WO 101

www.harcourt-international.com

Bringing you products from all Harcourt Health Sciences companies including Baillière Tindall, Churchill Livingstone, Mosby and W.B. Saunders

- ▶ **Browse** for latest information on new books, journals and electronic products

- ▶ **Search** for information on over 20 000 published titles with full product information including tables of contents and sample chapters

- ▶ **Keep up to date** with our extensive publishing programme in your field by registering with eAlert or requesting postal updates

- ▶ **Secure online ordering** with prompt delivery, as well as full contact details to order by phone, fax or post

- ▶ **News** of special features and promotions

If you are based in the following countries, please visit the country-specific site to receive full details of product availability and local ordering information

USA: www.harcourthealth.com

Canada: www.harcourtcanada.com

Australia: www.harcourt.com.au

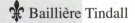 Baillière Tindall   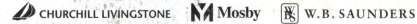 CHURCHILL LIVINGSTONE   Mosby   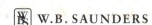 W.B. SAUNDERS

General Surgical Anatomy and Examination

Commissioning Editor: Laurence Hunter
Project Development Manager: Sarah Keer-Keer
Designer: Sarah Russell
Page make-up: Jim Farley
Project Controller: Nancy Arnott

General Surgical Anatomy and Examination

Alastair M. Thompson BSc (Hons) MD FRCSEd (Gen)

Reader and Honorary Consultant Surgeon
Department of Surgery,
Ninewells Hospital,
Dundee

Illustrated by **Paul Richardson**

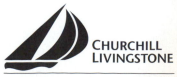
CHURCHILL
LIVINGSTONE

EDINBURGH LONDON NEW YORK PHILADELPHIA ST LOUIS SYDNEY TORONTO 2002

CHURCHILL LIVINGSTONE
An imprint of Harcourt Publishers Limited

© Harcourt Publishers Limited 2002

_D_ is a registered trademark of Harcourt Publishers Limited

First published 2002

ISBN 0443063761

International Student Edition ISBN 0443064636

British Library Cataloguing in Publication Data
A catalogue record for this book is available from the British Library

Library of Congress Cataloging in Publication Data
A catalog record for this book is available from the Library of Congress

Note
Medical knowledge is constantly changing. As new information becomes available, changes in treatment, procedures, equipment and the use of drugs become necessary. The author and the publishers have taken care to ensure that the information given in this text is accurate and up to date. However, readers are strongly advised to confirm that the information, especially with regard to drug usage, complies with the latest legislation and standards of practice.

The
publisher's
policy is to use
paper manufactured
from sustainable forests

Printed in Spain

Preface

The traditional, intensive and detailed anatomy training by dissection that occurs in the first year of medical school has often been largely forgotten by the time students reach their clinical years. By graduation, anatomy may be a distant memory. This book seeks to illustrate core anatomy and show its relevance to all those involved in the examination and history-taking of surgical patients.

This book does not seek to demonstrate every anatomical detail; there are excellent atlases which do just that. In real clinical practice, the human form has been subjected to many years of use and that is where recognition of key anatomical features is important in support of the history and examination.

This book is designed to facilitate comparison between normal and abnormal anatomy using body surface features and by use of radiological imaging. It should be used as a starting point to help understand how anatomy, clinical history and examination can be used to point to the diagnosis in patients with surgical conditions.

A.M.T   Dundee
                                         2002

Acknowledgements

This book has been inspired by the teaching of the anatomist Andrew Kerr of Edinburgh and the application of anatomy to surgical practice of the surgeon Alastair Munro of Inverness. I am indebted to Robert Wood of Dundee who provided so many of the colour slides in several chapters of this book; without his support this book would not have been possible. I am also grateful to David Smith and Rodney Mountain for slides of head and neck conditions, Robert Steele for the abdominal chapter and Peter Stonebridge for the lower limb images. The forbearance of patients and the Medical Media Department, Ninewells Hospital, Dundee at opportune moments has allowed this book to proceed.

The concepts that have been converted to the illustrated page in this book are a tribute to the vision and patience of Laurence Hunter, Sarah Keer-Keer, Alistair Christie and Paul Richardson.

Contents

1 Principles of examining the patient

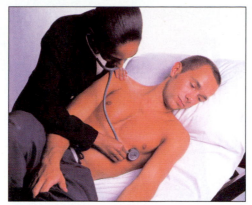

The anatomy of a living human varies from person to person. There are variations in the standard anatomy, size, shape and amount of fat padding between and around structures. The relationship of individual organs to the skin surface and to each other changes with movement (such as respiration) and with posture. While there are excellent atlases devoted to human anatomy, these are usually based on dissected specimens and may not relate deeper structures to the surface anatomy that you will examine in clinical practice. In addition, few texts seek to relate details of human anatomy to common surgical conditions. This book aims to bring together a core knowledge of normal anatomy and help relate this to disease processes by applying clinical history taking and examination techniques to general surgical patients. This should improve your diagnostic skills and help you understand the surgical approach when operating on patients.

Approach to the patient

Whatever problem a patient presents with, it is important to introduce yourself before you take a history, examine or investigate them (Table 1.1). You may know the patient's name and a few details, but he or she probably does not know who you are. Introducing yourself, shaking hands as you do so, establishes contact with the individual and can reduce some of the anxieties that a patient may have about the unfamiliar medical environment. This will make subsequent history taking and clinical examination of the patient much easier. Questioning and examining an anxious, tense person yields much less information than when he or she is more relaxed. It is both courteous and in some countries a legal obligation to seek the patient's permission to ask questions and subsequently examine them. A chaperone is advisable, particularly for male students and doctors when examining a female patient.

Fig. 1.1 Auscultating the heart

History
A patient's history comprises:
- the presenting complaint(s)
- history of the complaint(s)
- past medical, surgical and gynaecological history (including key questions on jaundice, rheumatic fever, tuberculosis, etc)
- medications and allergies
- social and family history
- alcohol and tobacco usage
- systematic enquiries regarding the cardiovascular, respiratory, gastrointestinal, genitourinary, neurological and musculoskeletal systems.

Examination
Ideally, a clinical examination should be conducted in a quiet, private setting. During examination, the region of the patient to be examined should be adequately exposed and the patient comfortable (Fig. 1.1). For the abdomen, this means exposing the patient from nipple to groin in a warm room with the patient lying flat, arms by their side, head placed on a single pillow. The bed the patient lies on should be at a height where you can comfortably inspect, palpate, percuss and auscultate the patient. A comfortable and relaxed patient and clinician can more easily relate the normal intra-abdominal anatomy (Fig. 1.2) to the detection of conditions suggested by the history. Care is always required to ensure as little as possible is missed.

Table 1.1 Approach to the patient	
Introduction	Palpation
Permission	Percussion
History	Auscultation
Exposure	Investigation
Positioning	Diagnosis
Inspection	Treatment

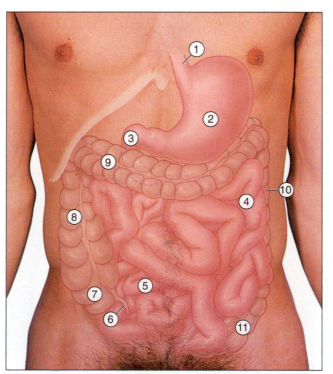

KEY
1. Oesophagus
2. Stomach
3. Duodenum
4. Jejunum
5. Ileum
6. Appendix
7. Caecum
8. Ascending colon
9. Transverse colon
10. Descending colon
11. Sigmoid colon

Fig. 1.2 Intra-abdominal anatomy related to the body surface

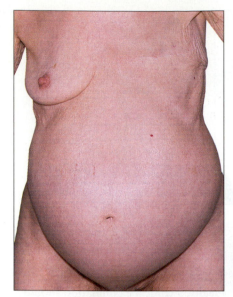

Fig. 1.3 Look for abdominal distension or asymmetry and ask about the cause of any visible scars

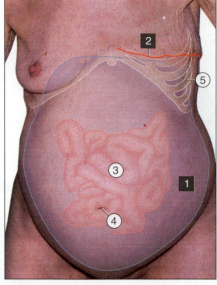

KEY

1. Distended abdomen (fluid, dull to percussion)
2. Mastectomy scar
3. Bowel (resonant to percussion)
4. Umbilicus
5. Ribs

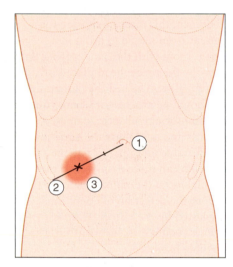

KEY

1. Umbilicus
2. Anterior supine thoracic spine *sup. ischiadic*
3. X = McBurney's point

Fig. 1.4 The site and extent of a painful or tender area suggests the underlying pathology. Such areas should be examined last, letting you examine the rest of the body before the patient tenses up as a reflex against stimulation of painful structures

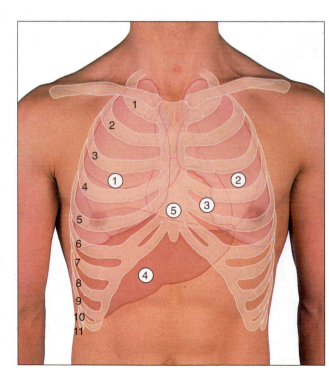

KEY

1. Right lung
2. Left lung
3. Heart
4. Liver
5. Sternum

Numbers 1–11 – ribs

Fig. 1.5 Normal anatomy of the chest related to the body surface

Inspection. This should include skin creases and the margins of the region exposed in order to be sure nothing is missed. Standing back and looking at the patient from the foot of the bed may well allow you to assess the general demeanour of the patient (e.g. jaundice) and detect distension 1, asymmetry or masses, particularly in the abdomen and groin (Fig. 1.3). It may be helpful to ask the patient about any visible scars 2.

Palpation. Before palpating any part of the body, remember to ask the patient if and where they are tender and where the pain radiates to (Fig. 1.4). Avoiding the tender area for as long as possible, and being as gentle as you can, is more comfortable for the patient. This lets you get information from your fingertips (such as feeling a mass) before the patient tenses up as a reflex against stimulation of painful structures. If there are paired structures (e.g. testes or breasts) examining the normal side first reinforces your knowledge of the patient's normal anatomy, but also reassures the patient how gentle and confident you are in your approach.

Percussion. This is particularly useful over the chest and abdomen, and here knowledge of the normal anatomy is vital. For example, remember the extent of the abdominal cavity under the ribcage (Fig. 1.5). Otherwise, one can be misled that the difference between the right and left side is due to intrathoracic pathology, whereas it is actually due to the liver 4 which lies deep to the right lower chest. The quality of the percussion note (e.g. tympanic, stony dull) and any differences between the right and left sides are key findings.

Auscultation. On auscultation, the correct use of a stethoscope's diaphragm or bell, placed in the best position, in quiet surroundings, will give the most information. Patient positioning (particularly when listening for heart sounds) and the radiation of sounds should be interpreted using your knowledge of the underlying anatomy.

Diagnosis

A differential diagnosis based on the history and clinical examination can then be further refined using investigations selected carefully from a standard list (Table 1.2). These should be chosen to give clinically useful information for the diagnosis and in preparing the patient for surgery, but avoiding unnecessary tests. Thus an ECG and chest radiograph are useful to help document the fitness of a 70-year-old smoker due to have an inguinal hernia repair.

Some structures are close to the skin surface and need only a little guidance as to how the pathology relates to the patient (Fig. 1.6). Other structures, particularly those buried in the chest or abdomen, are less easily visualized from the surface. They may require imaging to relate the pathological process to the patient's anatomy (Fig. 1.7). Where appropriate, the internal appearance (for example from endoscopic examination) or the pathology appearance following biopsy or resection is useful to establish the diagnosis and support a treatment plan. The definitive diagnosis for a patient is usually made on the basis of the history, examination and investigations prior to surgical intervention, where an operation is appropriate. Diagnosis at the time of operation is unusual, but can happen despite careful clinical appraisal and modern technology, particularly with intra-abdominal pathologies.

There is no substitute for seeing, examining and investigating as many patients as possible when you are a student, to hone your clinical and diagnostic skills. As a practising clinician you will continue to develop and refine these skills. This book should lay the foundation for you to relate symptoms and signs to the normal and abnormal anatomy of the patients you look after.

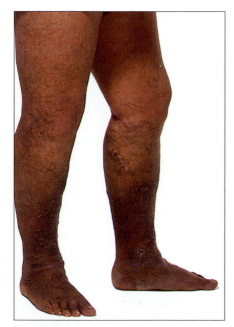

Fig. 1.6 Structures such as varicose veins lie close to the skin surface and it is easy to understand how the underlying condition relates to the patient's anatomy

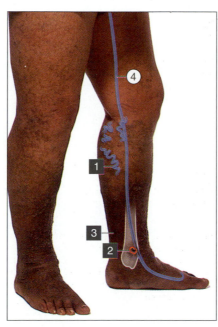

KEY

1	Varicosities	3	Skin discoloration
2	Varicose ulcer	4	Great saphenous vein

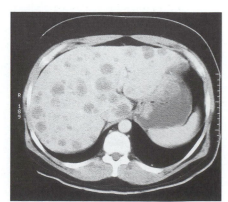

Fig. 1.7 Imaging techniques can reveal deeply buried pathology that is not detectable on simple clinical examination. This CT scan of the abdomen shows multiple metastases in the liver from a gastric cancer

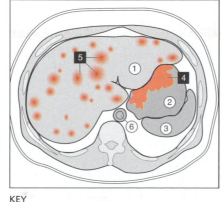

KEY

1	Liver	4	Gastric cancer
2	Stomach	5	Liver metastases
3	Spleen	6	Aorta

Table 1.2 Further investigations	
Urine dipstick test	Biochemistry/ microbiology
	Pregnancy test
Faeces	Occult blood Microbiology Tests of gastrointestinal function
Blood tests, including:	Haematology, coagulation Biochemistry Microbiology Immunology Blood transfusion Hormone levels
Cardiology	ECG Echocardiography
Radiology	Skull and cervical spine radiograph Chest radiograph Abdominal/pelvic radiograph Limb radiograph Contrast studies of: – gastrointestinal tract – vascular tree – urological system Ultrasound and Doppler scanning Computed tomography Magnetic resonance imaging Radionuclide imaging
Surgical studies	Proctoscopy Rigid sigmoidoscopy Upper endoscopy Flexible sigmoidoscopy/ colonoscopy Endoscopic retrograde cholangiopancreatography (ERCP)
Physiological studies	Upper gastrointestinal tract Lower gastrointestinal tract Urinary system Nervous system
Pathology	Cytology Biopsy

2 Head and neck

The neck is divided into a series of muscular triangles based on the muscles and bones of the cervical region (Fig. 2.1). The posterior triangle comprises the occipital ① and suprascapular ② triangles and the anterior triangle comprises the digastric ③ and carotid ④ triangles.

History

The clinical history for conditions of the head and neck should reflect the common pathological processes and conditions that affect this region (Table 2.1). The patient's age, local symptoms and systemic symptoms together with the examination findings will often suggest a differential diagnosis before confirmation of the diagnosis by investigations.

Local symptoms. If the patient presents with a swelling, ask about its position, size, shape, colour; tenderness, redness, discharge; duration, change in size; whether it is cystic or solid; and its relationship to eating or swallowing.

Systemic symptoms. Ask about symptoms suggestive of hyper-thyroidism (sweating, tremor, irritability, palpitations, weight loss) or hypothyroidism (cold intolerance, lethargy, change in voice), sweating or fevers (lymphoma, tuberculosis, viraemia, bacteraemia).

Past medical history. Smoking, alcohol intake, and exposure to radiation (particularly sunlight, radiotherapy treatment) are associated with carcinomas of the head and neck.

Medications may indicate the diagnosis, e.g. thyroxine for hypo-thyroidism, or any concomitant disease.

Family and social history. Family history may include a history of thyroid disease, or malignancy (if so, where?).

Social history should include travel, contact with animals (domestic or farm), contact with known disease carriers, racial origin and home circumstances.

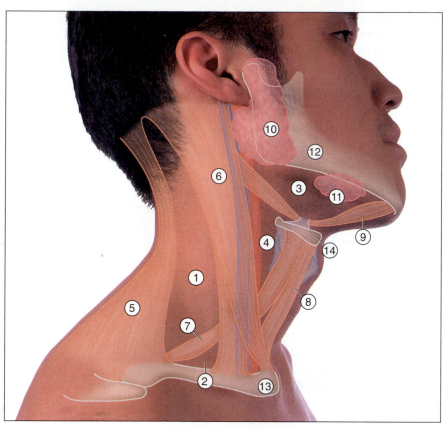

Fig. 2.1 Bony and muscular anatomy of the neck

KEY
① Occipital triangle
② Suprascapular triangle
③ Digastric triangle
④ Carotid triangle
⑤ Trapezius muscle
⑥ Sternocleidomastoid muscle
⑦ Omohyoid muscle
⑧ Sternohyoid muscle
⑨ Digastric muscle
⑩ Parotid gland
⑪ Submandibular gland
⑫ Mandible
⑬ Clavicle
⑭ Hyoid bone

Table 2.1 Differential diagnosis of head and neck lesions			
Congenital	Branchial cyst/branchial fistula (Fig. 2.20) Thyroglossal cyst (Fig. 2.21) Cystic hygroma (Fig. 2.22) Dermoid cyst Cervical rib		
Acquired	Reticuloendothelial	lymph node enlargement	Local (Fig. 2.7) Regional (Fig. 2.5) Generalized
	Gastrointestinal	Salivary gland enlargement	Parotid (Fig. 2.11) Submandibular (Fig. 2.12)
	Endocrine	Thyroid	Diffuse goitre (Fig. 2.14) Solitary nodule (Fig. 2.18) Multinodular goitre (Fig. 2.17)
	Skin	Basal cell carcinoma Squamous cell carcinoma (Fig. 2.9) Melanoma (Fig. 2.8) Sebaceous cyst (Fig. 10.1) Lipoma (Fig. 10.2)	

Examination

Exposure. Ensure that there is complete exposure of the head and neck down to the clavicles and that the hair does not obscure any part of the head and neck which you wish to examine. It is usually most comfortable for the patient and the clinician performing the examination to inspect the neck from the front (Figs 2.2, 2.4) and side (Fig. 2.3) and then to stand behind the seated patient to palpate the neck.

Inspection. From in front of the patient, inspect the head and neck for visible abnormalities and scars; take care to look for lesions or scars hidden in the skin lines or hairline, behind the ears or in the buccal cavity, if indicated by the history. Look for asymmetry between the right and left sides and for tracheal deviation.

If you are considering a thyroid (Fig. 2.2 ①, Fig. 2.4 **1** **2**) or midline neck swelling, you should ask the patient to swallow (easier with a cup of water) and look for upwards movement of the lump. If you suspect a facial palsy (following salivary gland surgery), ask the patient to whistle, then show their teeth, then screw up their eyes, movements which require an intact motor nerve (VII, facial nerve) to the facial muscles. Inspect eye movements, looking for lid lag/lid retraction, proptosis, chemosis (oedema of the cornea) in thyroid disease.

When inspecting for a lateral swelling (which may be bilateral) remember the extensive network of cervical lymph nodes (Fig. 2.3). These drain adjacent structures (e.g. submandibular nodes ⑥ drain the submandibular gland ⑲) which in turn drain to the deep cervical chain ④ and jugulodigastric node ⑤ around the internal jugular vein.

Palpation. Anterior structures (Fig. 2.2) such as the thyroid gland ①, anterior and posterior triangles of the neck, and supraclavicular fossae ⑪ are best palpated from behind, whereas the trachea ④ and some other midline structures are best palpated from in front, as also are the occipital lymph nodes (Fig. 2.3 ③).

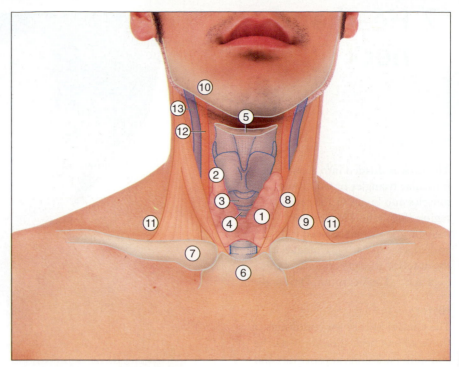

Fig. 2.2 Anterior aspect of the neck: bones, muscles, larynx and thyroid gland

KEY
① Thyroid gland
② Thyroid cartilage
③ Cricoid cartilage
④ First tracheal ring
⑤ Hyoid bone
⑥ Sternum
⑦ Clavicle
⑧ Sternocleidomastoid muscle – sternal head
⑨ Sternocleidomastoid muscle – clavicular head
⑩ Mandible
⑪ Supraclavicular fossae
⑫ Carotid artery
⑬ Internal jugular vein

Having asked whether any visible lesion is tender, aim to palpate a lump to measure the size (preferably with calipers) and reassess the shape, position and fixity relative to adjacent structures. Is the lump tethered or fixed to skin or underlying structures, or is it freely mobile? On palpation, does the lump move on swallowing? Is the lump pulsatile, expansile or fluctuant? (Use two fingers from one hand to fix the lump in position and a third digit to press gently between the other two to test for fluctuance.) Can the lump be transilluminated? If so, it is fluid filled. Are there any associated lumps such as palpable lymph nodes (Fig. 2.3)?

Buccal examination, palpating structures from within the oral cavity (such as salivary glands and ducts), should be performed using gloves to protect both the patient and examiner.

Percussion. Percussion over the thyroid and manubrium sternum (Fig. 2.2 ① and ⑥) may be used to try to confirm a retrosternal thyroid.

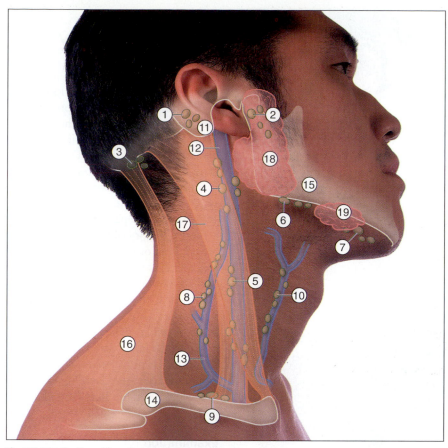

Fig. 2.3 Distribution of lymph nodes in the neck

KEY
1. Postauricular
2. Preauricular
3. Occipital
4. Deep cervical chain
5. Jugulodigastric node
6. Submandibular
7. Submental
8. Superficial cervical chain
9. Supraclavicular
10. Superficial cervical chain around anterior jugular veins
11. Mastoid bone
12. Internal jugular vein
13. External jugular vein
14. Clavicle
15. Mandible
16. Trapezius
17. Sternocleidomastoid muscle
18. Parotid gland
19. Submandibular gland

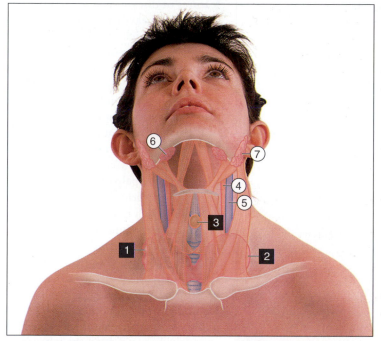

Fig. 2.4 Thyroid gland abnormalities in the neck

KEY
1. Multinodular thyroid goitre
2. Diffuse goitre
3. Thyroglossal cyst
4. Carotid artery
5. Internal jugular vein
6. Submandibular gland
7. Parotid gland

Auscultation. When auscultating over the carotid arteries (Fig. 2.4 ④) for a bruit, the bruit may be most easily heard when the patient holds his breath. Listen to both sides and be aware that an occluded artery may have no blood flow and hence no bruit, and that an aortic murmur may be transmitted to the neck. A bruit may (rarely) be palpable over a hypervascular goitre 1 2 as a thrill.

Investigations.

- Full blood count for anaemia, elevated white cell count
- Monospot test (for Epstein–Barr virus infection)
- Plasma viscosity or erythrocyte sedimentation rate
- Blood biochemistry, liver function tests, proteins
- TSH for thyroid status (with free T_3 and T_4 if TSH is abnormal)
- Ultrasound for lumps in the head and neck to determine whether they are solid or cystic and which structures they relate to
- Fine needle aspiration using a 19 gauge needle to aspirate a cystic lump or to aspirate a solid lump for diagnostic cytopathological examination
- Core/incisional/excisional biopsy to establish a tissue diagnosis.

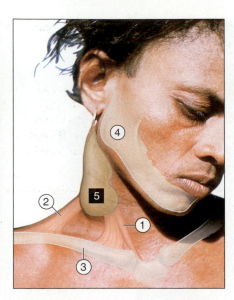

Fig. 2.5 Swollen jugulodigastric nodes

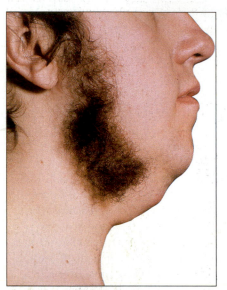

Fig. 2.6 Swollen submandibular nodes

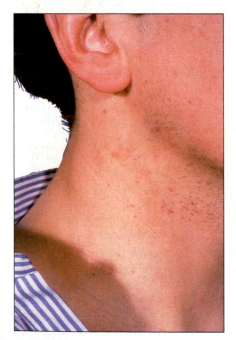

Fig. 2.7 Swollen posterior triangle node

Cervical lymphadenopathy

History

Ask about the number, position (Fig. 2.3), duration and any discomfort in the nodes. Are there any other lesions in the head and neck (see Figs 2.8, 2.9), or within the mouth (see Fig. 2.13), from which the nodes could be draining? Have there been any systemic symptoms, e.g. sweating, malaise, anorexia? In the past medical history, is there a history of malignancy (e.g. breast, lung or intra-abdominal cancer)? Has there been any travel abroad or contact with people with illness, or with animals? Are there lumps elsewhere in the body (e.g. groin or axilla)? The age of the patient may suggest likely diagnoses – infections (viral or bacterial) are more common in younger people, whereas malignancy is more likely in older people.

Examination

On inspection, look for any general features of disease such as jaundice or cachexia or heavily nicotine-stained fingers. See which lymph nodes are visible – comment on their position and whether they are single (Fig. 2.7 [7]) or multiple (Figs 2.5 [5], 2.6 [6]). Look inside the mouth for intraoral causes of lymphadenopathy (Fig. 2.13).

On palpation, standing behind the patient, palpate both sides simultaneously to allow comparison. Systematically palpate the node groups to confirm their position and ascertain which nodes are involved. Start with the submental nodes, palpating the submandibular region (Fig. 2.6 [6]), then the preauricular region, then down through the anterior triangle, including the jugulodigastric nodes (Fig. 2.5 [5]) and the nodes between the heads of sternocleidomastoid (on the left side

KEY
1. Sternocleidomastoid muscle
2. Trapezius muscle
3. Clavicle
4. Mandible
5. Jugulodigastric nodes
6. Submandibular nodes
7. Posterior triangle node

known as Virchow's node). Passing laterally, via infraclavicular fossa nodes, pass into the posterior triangle (Fig. 2.7) feeling for supraclavicular fossa nodes, then superiorly up to the retroauricular and occipital nodes. Are the nodes single (Fig. 2.7) or multiple (Fig. 2.6) or matted (Fig. 2.5); fixed to skin or underlying structures; soft, rubbery or hard? Record your findings in diagrammatic form.

Investigation and treatment
A full blood count, blood film and ESR/plasma viscosity may be supplemented by viral titres, monospot test for EBV, and testing for TB and other organisms (e.g. actinomycosis).

Chest radiology may show an intrathoracic lesion (bronchogenic carcinoma, secondary malignancy, TB). Ultrasound examination of the neck, endoscopy, fine needle aspiration cytology or surgical biopsy of the palpable lymph node will suggest the dignosis and treatment for the lymphadenopathy.

Squamous cell carcinoma and melanoma

Skin cancers (basal cell carcinoma, squamous cell carcinoma and melanoma) are comparatively common in the head and neck because these areas are exposed to more sunlight.

History and examination
Ask the patient's age, about exposure to sunlight, occupation and any previous history of skin lesions. A melanoma (Table 2.2) may arise from a previous pigmented skin lesion. Ask about a change in **size**, **shape** or **colour**, which are the three most common symptoms. Itch and bleeding may also occur. Note the site, duration of the change in a lesion and any additional similar lesions or lumps. A clinical photograph (Fig. 2.8) may be useful to document the features of the melanoma **1** .

A squamous cell carcinoma (Fig. 2.9) presents as an enlarging skin lesion, which may bleed and form a crust. Ask about any associated lumps **8** **9** **10** in the neck, their location and their duration.

On inspection, note the position of the lesion, the size (measured in mm using calipers), colour, shape and contour. Look for the presence of satellite lesions or more distant metastatic spread (to regional lymph nodes, or to the liver, for example,

causing jaundice).

On palpation, examine the regional lymph nodes and liver for enlargement.

Investigation and treatment
Investigation may include excisional biopsy of the lesion and fine needle aspiration cytology of the regional lymph nodes if metastatic disease is suspected.

Treatment for melanoma is by excision including a 1 cm margin of normal skin with appropriate reconstructive surgery to the site of the melanoma. Metastatic lymph nodes may be excised and a range of chemotherapies may be used.

Prognosis depends on the depth of invasion of the melanoma (Table 2.3).

Treatment of squamous cell carcinoma may involve surgical excision and/or radiotherapy.

Table 2.2 Classification of melanomas

- Lentigo maligna melanoma
- Superficial spreading
- Acral lentiginous (on the sole or palm)
- Subungual
- Nodular

Table 2.3 Breslow scale for melanoma

Breslow thickness	5-year survival rate
1.5 mm	90%
1.5–3 mm	60%
3.5 mm	<50%

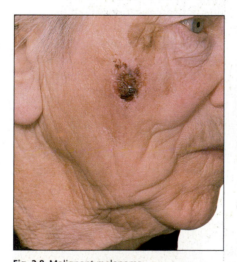

Fig. 2.8 Malignant melanoma

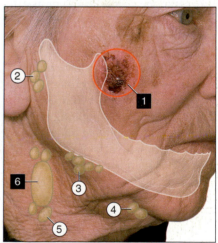

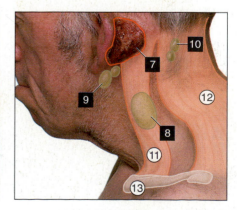

Fig. 2.9 Squamous cell carcinoma

KEY
1. Lentigo malignant melanoma
2. Preauricular nodes
3. Submandibular nodes
4. Submental nodes
5. Deep cervical chain
6. Enlarged jugulodigastric node
7. Squamous carcinoma
8. Metastatic jugulodigastric node
9. Metastatic postauricular nodes
10. Metastatic occipital nodes
11. Sternocleidomastoid muscle
12. Trapezius muscle
13. Clavicle

Parotid salivary glands

The parotid glands each have a deep (retromandibular) and superficial (preauricular) lobe intimately related to the facial nerve (VIIth cranial nerve) (Fig. 2.10). The parotid glands are commonly affected by infection (mumps), autoimmune disease (e.g. Sjögren's syndrome), tumours (see Table 2.4) or stones.

History

Ask about the duration of the swelling, whether it is unilateral or bilateral, painful or tender on palpation, or increases in size with salivary stimulation (suggesting a duct stone). Ask about systemic symptoms, such as prodromal illness, and symptoms suggestive of connective tissue disease such as joint or muscle pains, dry eyes or dry mouth.

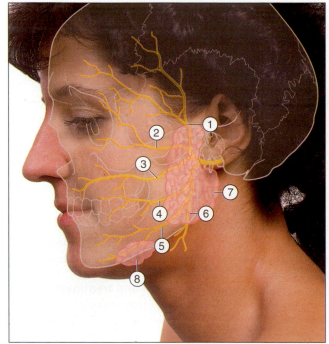

KEY
1. Temporal
2. Zygomatic
3. Upper buccal
4. Lower buccal
5. Marginal mandibular
6. Communicating with transverse cutaneous nerve of neck
7. Parotid gland
8. Submandibular gland

Fig. 2.10 Facial nerve and major salivary glands of head and neck

Examination

Inspection. Look for symmetry of the right and left sides – are both parotids or just one gland enlarged; if so is it the whole gland or only the superficial portion? Inspect for VIIth cranial nerve (facial) palsy, either as a consequence of the pathological process in the parotid gland or as a consequence of surgery to the gland with subsequent nerve damage (see Fig. 2.10 for normal anatomy).

Palpation. Before palpating the parotid gland remember to ask if the gland is tender. Palpate from behind the patient, gently comparing right with left and attempting to delineate whether the superficial (Fig. 2.11 **1**), deep **2** or both parts of the gland are enlarged.

Remember to inspect and palpate inside the mouth (wearing gloves) – the parotid duct orifice opens opposite the second upper molar tooth and a stone may be visible or palpable in the duct.

Palpate the regional lymph nodes, including the preauricular, retroauricular, cervical and occipital nodes for metastatic spread.

Investigation

A raised white cell count or lymphocytosis may be demonstrated in response to viral infection of the parotid. Autoimmune antibodies should be measured if a systemic autoimmune condition is suspected. Ultrasound of the gland may demonstrate the anatomy of the parotid gland and abnormal structures within it such as a tumour (Fig. 2.11 **1**). Fine needle aspiration cytology or core biopsy (under local anaesthesia) may confirm the diagnosis.

Treatment

Treatment of viral parotitis is expectant. Treatment of tumours of the parotid is by excision, avoiding nerve damage, and radiotherapy.

Table 2.4 Tumours of the parotid gland	
Type of lesion	**Features**
Pleomorphic adenomas	Most commonly in parotid. Benign/slow growth, but local recurrence if enucleated Patients usually <50 years of age
Adenolymphoma	Often soft/partially cystic Benign/slow growing Patients usually >50 years of age
Anaplastic carcinoma	Fast growing Hard and woody Invades locally VIIth cranial nerve palsy Regional lymphadenopathy Retrotonsillar enlargement

KEY
1. Superficial parotid
2. Deep parotid
3. Mandible
4. Sternocleidomastoid muscle
5. Facial nerve

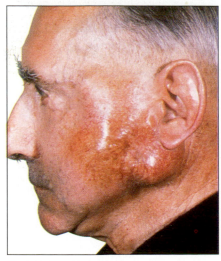
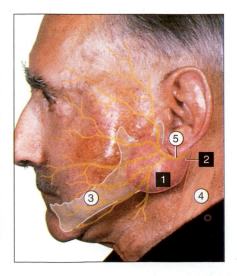

Fig. 2.11 Parotid gland tumour

Submandibular salivary glands

The submandibular gland is more frequently the site of stone formation and less frequently the site of tumour than the parotid gland (Table 2.4). The submandibular gland may be difficult to distinguish clinically from submandibular lymph nodes and even from lesions in the floor of the mouth. It also has superficial and deep components and the duct opens near the midline in the floor of the mouth.

History

Ask about the duration of salivary gland swelling, whether it is unilateral (Fig. 2.12 **1**) or bilateral, painful or tender on palpation, increases in size with salivary stimulation (such as at meal times) and discharges saliva with subsequent resolution of the swelling (suggesting a duct stone). Also ask about systemic symptoms, such as a prodromal illness or symptoms suggestive of connective tissue disease.

Examination

On inspection, compare the two sides externally (Fig. 2.12) and on inspecting the floor of the mouth look to see if there is a stone obstructing the duct.

Palpation. Ask first if there is any discomfort and gently commence palpation externally in the submental region, palpating the submandibular region with the pulps of your fingers as they pass posteriorly. Usually the patient tries to be helpful by raising the chin; this has the opposite effect of tightening the musculature, which makes palpation more difficult, so ask the patient to gently drop his head forwards. Palpate for regional lymphadenopathy in the anterior triangle nodes, the jugulodigastric nodes and deep cervical chain of nodes.

Remember to use gloved fingers to palpate inside the floor of the mouth, for which bimanual palpation (one finger inside the mouth, the other hand outside in the submandibular region) can be very helpful.

Investigations

Ultrasound scanning of a submandibular swelling has largely superseded plain radiology of the floor of the mouth or sialography to detect a stone, and may show other pathological processes. Fine needle aspiration cytology or core biopsy (under anaesthetic) may confirm the diagnosis.

Treatment

A symptomatic gland may settle with time, but surgical excision is required if tumour is suspected.

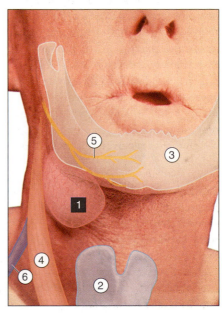

Fig. 2.12 Swollen submandibular gland

KEY
1 Submandibular gland
(2) Thyroid cartilage
(3) Mandible
(4) Sternocleidomastoid muscle
(5) Marginal mandibular branch of facial nerve
(6) External jugular vein

Intraoral lesions

An intraoral lesion such as a squamous carcinoma of the tongue (Fig. 2.13 **1**) will only be evident if you ask the patient to stick out his tongue and look inside the mouth. Assess the position, size and colour of the lesion and palpate for lymph nodes in the submental, submandibular and cervical chains (see Fig. 2.3).

Following biopsy, treatment is by surgical excision and/or radiotherapy.

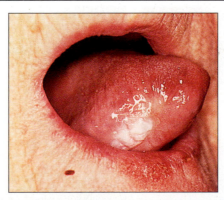

Fig. 2.13 Squamous cancer of the tongue

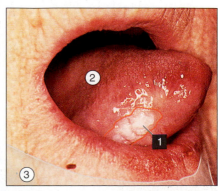

KEY
1 Squamous cancer
(2) Tongue
(3) Mandible

Thyroid gland

History

Age and place of residence may suggest the likely cause of a thyroid neck lump. Ask whether the lump is unilateral or bilateral (Figs 2.14, 2.17), a single, multiple or diffuse swelling, tender (goitres are usually painless but thyroiditis, haemorrhage into a cyst or carcinoma may cause pain) or non-tender. What is it's duration and has there been any change in size?

Ask about symptoms of hyperthyroidism (sweating, agitation, tremor, irritability, palpitations, weight loss, heat intolerance, diarrhoea) or hypothyroidism (lethargy, weight gain, cold intolerance, change in voice, menstrual disturbance). A large (Fig. 2.17 **1**) or retrosternal (Fig. 2.16 **4**) thyroid may cause stridor due to tracheal compression and an anaplastic carcinoma may cause hoarseness and a bovine cough due to recurrent laryngeal nerve palsy.

Examination

Inspection. Look for eye and skin signs of thyroid disease:

- for hyperthyroidism (Fig. 2.15) – proptosis, lid retraction, lid lag, corneal oedema (chemosis), warm periphery, sweating skin, fine hand tremor, and more rarely, ophthalmoplegia
- for hypothyroidism (Fig. 2.14) – coarse features, periorbital puffiness, dry skin and thinned hair.

On inspection from the front of the patient, look to see if the thyroid has a unilateral or bilateral swelling (Fig. 2.14 **1**, 2.17 **1**), and appears to be diffuse or nodular. Ask the patient to swallow to confirm that the swelling moves up then down with swallowing (the thyroid is invested by the pretracheal fascia so moves on swallowing). See whether the trachea is central.

On palpation, ask first if the neck is tender, then, standing behind the patient, gently palpate both left and right lobes of the thyroid, feeling for lumps or diffuse smoothness and ask the patient to swallow, demonstrating that the palpable thyroid moves. Is the thyroid hard and woody (associated with malignancy or thyroiditis) or soft? Is there fixation to the trachea?

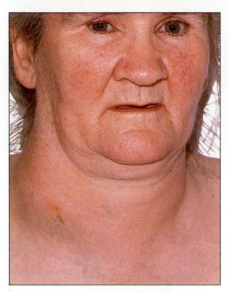

Fig. 2.14 Woman with bilateral goitre

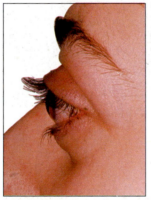

Fig. 2.15 Appearance of the eyes in hyperthyroidism – proptosis, lid retraction, chemosis

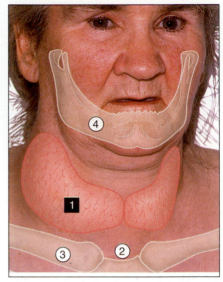

KEY
1 Diffuse goitre
② Sternal notch
③ Clavicle
④ Mandible

KEY
① Clavicle
② First rib
3 Goitre
4 Retrosternal goitre
⑤ Arch of aorta
⑥ Manubrium sternum

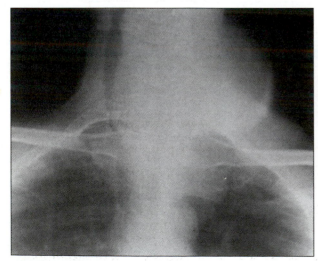

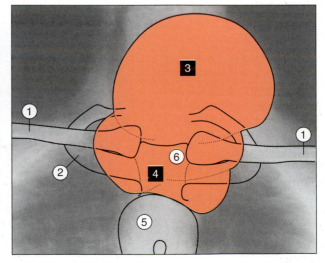

Fig. 2.16 Radiograph of retrosternal goitre

Palpate for regional lymphadenopathy.

On percussion over the sternum, is there dullness suggestive of retrosternal goitre (Fig. 2.16 4)? Limb reflexes may be enhanced in hyperthyroidism or slow in hypothyroidism.

On auscultation over the thyroid gland, listen for the bruit of hyperdynamic blood flow through a thyroid affected by Graves' disease.

Investigation

TSH is used to determine whether a patient is hypothyroid (raised TSH), hyperthyroid (low TSH) or euthyroid (normal TSH), findings which can be confirmed by measuring T_3/T_4 if necessary. If Hashimoto's thyroiditis or Graves' disease is suspected, then circulating antithyroid antibodies and thyroid-stimulating immunoglobulins can be measured, and in medullary carcinoma, calcitonin is raised. A chest radiograph supplemented by thoracic outlet views may demonstrate a retrosternal thyroid (Fig. 2.16), but ultrasound is most useful to determine whether a thyroid swelling is solid, cystic, single, multiple or diffuse. Fine needle aspiration of a cyst or solid lump in the thyroid can be diagnostic and (for a cyst) therapeutic. Radionuclide scanning (Fig. 2.18) is still used in some centres to determine whether a single lump is 'cold' – has lower uptake than the surrounding thyroid (Fig 2.18 1) (hence likely to be malignant), or 'hot' – with increased uptake relative to the surrounding thyroid (hence functional and benign).

Treatment

Treatment depends on the underlying pathology of the thyroid swelling (Fig. 2.19) and the thyroid status of the patient. The treatment may be conservative (for benign minimally enlarged euthyroid goitre), medical (dietary iodine, replacement of thyroxin in hypothyroidism or suppression of thyroid activity in hyperthyroidism), radioiodine or surgical resection (thyroid lobectomy, subtotal or total thyroidectomy) depending on the specific pathology. Rare surgical complications include recurrent laryngeal nerve palsy, superior laryngeal nerve palsy, hypocalcaemia (due to parathyroid damage) or tracheal compression due to haematoma.

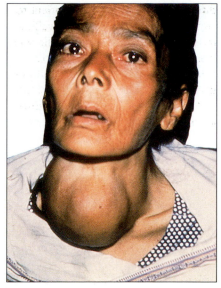
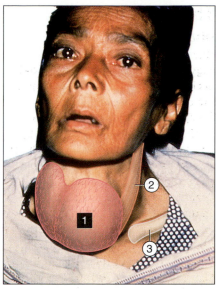

Fig. 2.17 Multinodular goitre with dominant nodule

Key
1 Goitre with dominant nodule
2 Sternocleidomastoid muscle
3 Clavicle

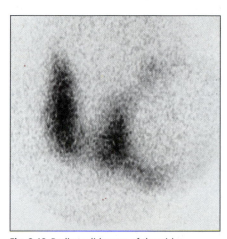
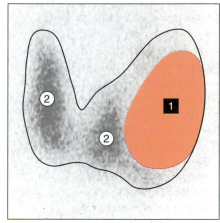

Fig. 2.18 Radionuclide scan of thyroid

Key
1 'Cold nodule'
2 Normal thyroid

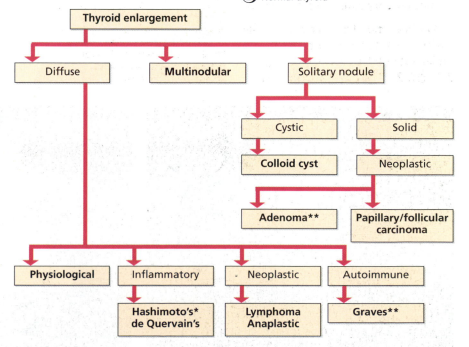

Fig. 2.19 Thyroid swellings (* may be associated with hypothyroidism, ** may be associated with hyperthyropidism)

Congenital neck swellings

Branchial cyst/branchial fistula

A branchial cyst or fistula (Fig. 2.20) develops because of failure of fusion of the second and third branchial arches. Usually a cyst becomes notice- able during the second decade of life, as a swelling just deep to the middle third of the sternocleidomastoid muscle ①, which may be tender. A branchial fistula **8** communicates between the tonsillar fossa and the skin at the junction of the middle and lower thirds of the sternocleido- mastoid muscle **7** . Aspiration of the cyst will confirm the diagnosis, and excision of the cyst or fistula **8** can be performed.

Thyroglossal cyst

A thyroglossal cyst (Fig. 2.21 **9**) is an embryonic remnant of thyroid tissue in the midline of the neck superior to the isthmus of the gland, which also moves with swallowing and on protruding the tongue. It may be connected, via a remnant passing deep to the hyoid bone, to the foramen caecum at the base of the tongue.

Ultrasound will confirm the diagnosis and excision may remove the cyst.

Cystic hygroma

A cystic hygroma (a collection of dilated lymphatic channels) usually presents in early childhood as a soft, fluctuant, compressible, unilateral cystic swelling in the neck (Fig. 2.22 **10**), which should transilluminate.

Treatment is by excision.

KEY
① Sternocleidomastoid muscle
② Sternal notch
③ Mandible
④ Thyroid cartilage
⑤ Clavicle
⑥ Trachea
7 Site of fistula opening
8 Fistula tract
9 Thyroglossal cyst
10 Cystic hygroma

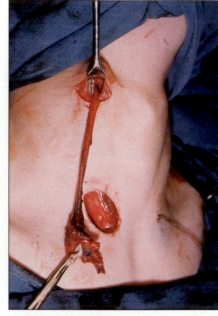
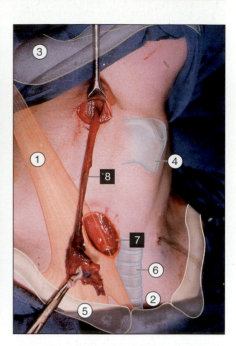

Fig. 2.20 Branchial fistula

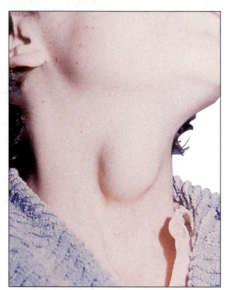

Fig. 2.21 Thyroglossal cyst

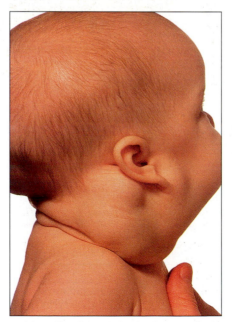
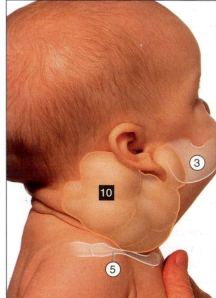

Fig. 2.22 Cystic hygroma in a baby

3 Chest

Respiratory and cardiac conditions commonly occur in patients undergoing surgery and as complications of surgery or surgical diseases.

History

The main respiratory symptoms are cough, sputum, haemoptysis, breathlessness (at rest, on exertion) chest pain (sharp, i.e. pleuritic) and wheeze. These symptoms may be caused by infections (pneumonia, empyema, bronchiectasis, tuberculosis), tumours (primary lung carcinoma, secondary pulmonary or pleural metastases), vascular problems (pulmonary embolism/infarction, heart failure) or trauma (fractured ribs).

The main cardiac symptoms are chest pain (gripping or crushing rather than sharp), breathlessness (on exertion, on lying flat or at rest), palpitations and ankle swelling.

Past medical history with regard to the chest should include previous thoracic or cardiac surgery, injuries, pneumothorax, rheumatic fever, tuberculosis; previous pneumonia, childhood measles or whooping cough; current and previous smoking habit (number of cigarettes), current medications (their indications, duration) and how often these are used.

Ask about a family history of respiratory or cardiovascular disease, and the patient's occupation (mining, working with asbestos, farming).

Examination

The clinical examination should be based on the normal anatomy (Fig. 3.1a and b) and aim to detect signs suggested by the history.

Examine the hands for finger clubbing (Fig. 3.2), splinter haemorrhages, leuconychia, palmar erythema and the radial pulse (see below); the head and neck for signs of central cyanosis of the lips and tongue, raised jugulovenous pressure and lymphadenopathy. There may be associated abdominal signs (such as hepatomegaly, ascites) or peripheral oedema.

The torso should be exposed to the waist to allow you to examine the front and the back, and compare the left and right sides.

Inspection. Observe the respiratory rate and which muscles are being used. Look for the presence of any deformities (kyphosis, scoliosis) and surgical scars. Inspect any sputum pot for the colour of sputum and/or the presence of blood.

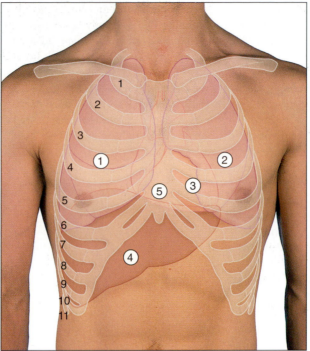

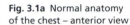

KEY
1. Right lung
2. Left lung
3. Heart
4. Liver
5. Sternum
6. Spine of 7th cervical vertebra
7. 12th thoracic vertebra
8. Scapula
Numbers 1–12 – ribs

Fig. 3.1a Normal anatomy of the chest – anterior view

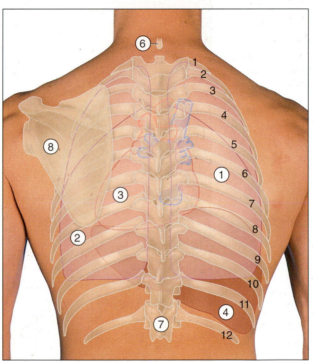

Fig. 3.1b Normal anatomy of the chest – posterior view

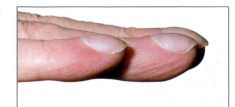

Fig. 3.2 Finger clubbing

Inspect for the presence of a cardiac pacemaker and listen for the clicking of prosthetic heart valves (Fig. 3.15).

With the patient propped up at 45 degrees, measure the jugulovenous pressure in cm above the sternal notch.

Palpation. Examine the position of the trachea for deviation to one side (pushed by intrathoracic expansion, pulled by collapse or contraction). Palpate for the apex beat, which may be displaced from its normal position in the fifth intercostal space in the midclavicular line, for thrills and for a parasternal heave.

Use the flat of your hand to test for chest expansion, and compare the right and left sides of the upper, mid and lower zones, both front and back.

Palpate with the flat of your hands for vocal fremitus: ask the patient to say '1–1–1' as you palpate each side, comparing right and left.

Percussion. Percuss the back, then the front of the chest comparing right with left. Progressively percuss the supraclavicular fossae, clavicles, first intercostal space working your way down the anterior chest wall and bearing in mind the upper (Fig. 3.3a ①), middle ② and lower ③ lobes on the right but upper ④ and lower ⑤ lobes on the left. Similar percussion of the posterior chest wall (Fig. 3.3b) will help you establish where the percussion note changes from resonant to dull.

Auscultation. Compare left with right anteriorly and posteriorly using a similar scheme to percussion.

Listen for breath sounds using the bell of the stethoscope:
• crepitations (fine/coarse, do they clear with coughing?)
• bronchial breathing over an area of consolidation
• whispering pectoriloquy for transmission of sound over the consolidated region (ask the patient to say '1–1–1').

Listen for a pleural rub over an area of pleuritis, which reflects a pathological process in the underlying lung.

Avoid listening within 3 cm of the midline where the sternum (anteriorly) and spinal muscles (posteriorly) impair auscultation.

Percussion and auscultation laterally (Fig. 3.4) may help in supplementing information gained from examining the anterior (Fig. 3.3a) and posterior (Fig. 3.3b) chest wall. On the right side, remember that the liver (Figs 3.3a ⑩ 3.4④) lies deep to the ribs with the diaphragm (Fig. 3.4⑧) surprisingly high on expiration.

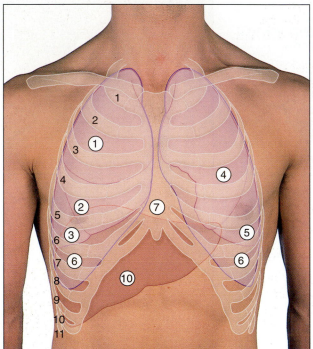

KEY
① Right upper lobe
② Right middle lobe
③ Right lower lobe
④ Left upper lobe
⑤ Left lower lobe
⑥ Pleural space
⑦ Sternum
⑧ Seventh cervical vertebra
⑨ Scapula
⑩ Liver
Numbers 1–11 – ribs

Fig. 3.3a Anterior view of the chest and ribs

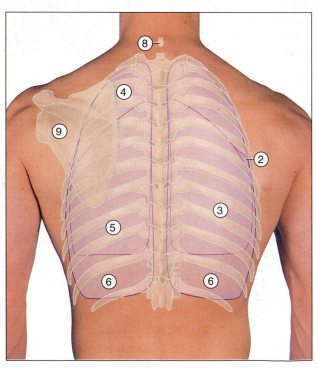

Fig. 3.3b Posterior view of the chest and ribs

Investigation

Haematology may show a raised white cell count and a raised ESR/plasma viscosity in an infective or inflammatory process, or anaemia as an exacerbating factor for cardio-respiratory symptoms. The pro-thrombin time ratio, or international normalized ratio, is used to monitor control of anticoagulation with warfarin (for example after pulmonary embolism).

Biochemistry may demonstrate electrolyte disturbances that can precipitate or worsen cardiac dys-rhythmias (particularly hypokalaemia, hyperkalaemia).

Measurement of arterial P_{O_2}, P_{CO_2} and acid–base balance may confirm the presence of hypoxia or hypercarbia and/or compensatory changes with metabolic or respiratory acidosis or alkalosis.

Urinary testing is indicated to detect glucose in diabetics and proteins in renal disease.

Chest radiography and CT scanning may be used to delineate an intrathoracic abnormality. A chest radiograph (or X-ray) (Fig. 3.5) is usually taken upright by placing the X-ray film against the anterior chest and shooting through the X-rays from the back (PA film) which minimizes magnification effects on the heart. This posteroanterior (PA) film may be supplemented by lateral views.

A 12 lead ECG will assess cardiac rate and rhythm, the presence of signs of current or previous myocardial damage and may show evidence of right heart strain following pulmonary embolism.

Spirometry may be used to measure the FEV_1, FVC, FEV_1/FVC ratio and more complex measures of respiratory function.

Sputum cytology, needle aspiration of a pleural effusion and bronchoscopy (perhaps with biopsy or lavage) can all be used to obtain a cytopathological diagnosis.

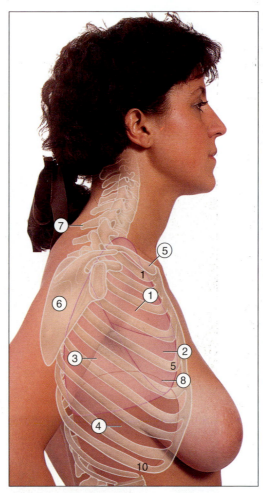

KEY
1. Upper right lobe
2. Middle lobe
3. Right lower lobe
4. Liver
5. Clavicle
6. Scapula
7. 7th cervical spinal process
8. Diaphragm

Numbers 1, 5 and 10 – ribs

Fig. 3.4 Lateral view of the chest

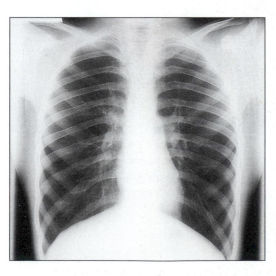

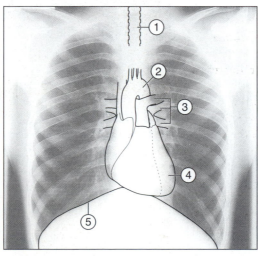

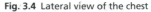

KEY
1. Trachea
2. Aortic arch
3. Pulmonary vessels
4. Left ventricle
5. Diaphragm

Fig. 3.5 Normal posteroanterior (PA) chest radiograph on deep inspiration

Pneumonia

History
Duration of cough and productivity (sputum, blood), smoking, enforced immobility due to other medical conditions, surgical operations, etc., pyrexia, sweating, travel abroad or proximity to animals, and chronic pulmonary conditions predisposing to pneumonia (e.g. chronic obstructive pulmonary disease) provide useful clues as to the likely underlying diagnosis.

Examination (Table 3.1)
On inspection, look for central cyanosis, increased respiratory rate, perspiration, an oxygen mask or a nebulizer.

On palpation, examine for clamminess, for tracheal deviation (Fig. 3.9) (towards pulmonary collapse and consolidation secondary to pneumonia) and chest expansion.

On percussion, listen for dullness over the affected lower, mid or upper zone (for lobar pneumonia) or the whole lung field (for broncho-pneumonia).

On auscultation, listen for bronchial breathing, crepitations (fine or more commonly coarse crackles) and wheeze (rhonchi) over the affected lung region (Figs 3.6 **1** , 3.7 **1**).

Investigations
Investigations include full blood count (for raised white cell count), plasma viscosity/ESR, arterial blood gases and chest radiography (Figs 3.6 and 3.7).

Treatment
Humidified oxygen, nebulized bronchodilators, physiotherapy and appropriate antibiotics (administered by the oral or intravenous route) are used in treatment. Exacerbating factors such as cigarette smoking should be stopped.

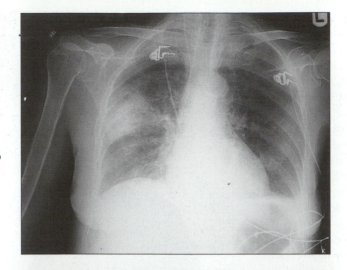

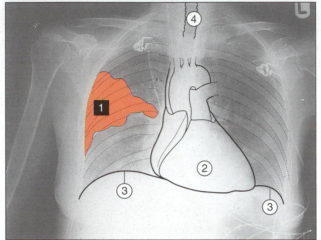

KEY
1. Middle lobe pneumonia
2. Heart and great vessels
3. Diaphragm
4. Trachea

Fig. 3.6 Posteroanterior (PA) chest radiograph of pneumonia

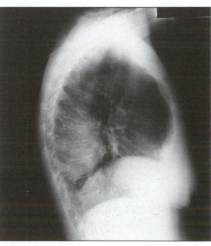

Fig. 3.7 Lateral radiograph of pneumonia

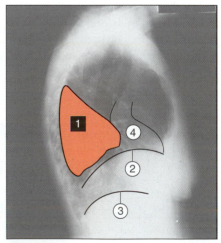

KEY
1. Middle lobe pneumonia
2. Right diaphragm
3. Left diaphragm
4. Heart

Table 3.1 Features of right middle lobe pneumonia		
	Right	**Left**
Chest expansion	? reduced	Normal
Percussion note	Dull over mid lobe	Normal
Breath sounds	Bronchial	Normal
Added sounds	Crepitations + rhonchi	Normal
Vocal resonance	Increased	Normal

Pneumothorax

History
Pay particular attention to a history of trauma (penetrating, such as a knife wound, or blunt, such as a road traffic accident or kick), or a history of previous spontaneous pneumo-thoraces. The key to detecting a pneumothorax is to remember it as a possible diagnosis.

Examination (Table 3.2)
Some signs may only be present in the presence of an acute (Fig. 3.8 **1**) or even tension (Fig. 3.9 **4**) pneumo-thorax.

On inspection, look for increased respiratory rate, tracheal deviation (Fig. 3.8 **2**), the hyperinflated appearance of the chest, and the presence of a bony trauma **4** or a chest drain.

On palpation, examine for tracheal deviation **2**, reduced expansion on the side of the chest with the pneumothorax, and absent vocal fremitus.

On percussion, compare right with left sides, seeking evidence of hyper-resonance of the pneumothorax **1** compared with the patient's normal chest.

On auscultation, listen for reduced or absent breath sounds over the side of the pneumothorax.

Investigations
A chest radiograph will show the presence of a pneumothorax (Fig. 3.8 **1**). Analysis of arterial blood gases will detect hypoxia if respiratory function is compromised.

Treatment
This is by aspiration or underwater sealed tube drainage of the pneumo-thorax if >20% of the lung field is affected or if the patient is symptomatic.

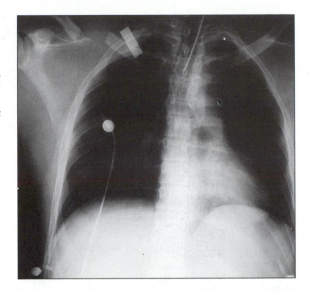

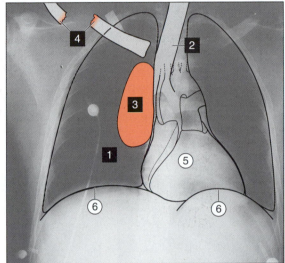

KEY

1	Acute pneumothorax
2	Trachea deviated to collapsed site
3	Collapsed lung
4	Fractured clavicle
⑤	Heart
⑥	Diaphragm

Fig. 3.8 Chest radiograph of pneumothorax

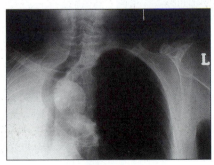

Fig. 3.9 Deviation of trachea

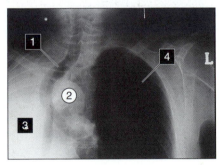

KEY

1	Trachea deviated to right
②	Aortic arch
3	Consolidated lung
4	Tension pneumothorax

Table 3.2 Features of right pneumothorax		
	Right	**Left**
Chest expansion	Reduced	Normal/reduced
Percussion note	Hyper-resonant	Normal
Breath sounds	Absent	Present, normal
Added sounds	None	None
Vocal resonance	None	Normal

Bronchial carcinoma

History
Ask about cough, haemoptysis, smoking, previous lung disease, and occupational exposure (miners).

Examination
On **inspection**, look for nicotine-stained fingers, finger clubbing (Fig. 3.2), cachexia. Less frequently encountered are skin metastases, superior vena caval obstruction (due to advanced mediastinal disease) or non-metastatic systemic effects. Listen for recurrent laryngeal nerve palsy (hoarseness).

On **palpation**, examine for tracheal deviation towards the side of the lesion, palpate for cervical lymph-adenopathy or hepatomegaly as signs of metastatic disease. Palpate for chest expansion.

On **percussion**, seek dullness over regions of collapse and consolidation (Fig. 3.10 **3**) distal to a bronchogenic carcinoma **2** , or stony dullness at the lower zone secondary to a pleural effusion **4** . Compare right and left for evidence of unilateral or bilateral pleural effusion **4** .

On **auscultation**, listen for crackles or wheeze associated with regions of collapse **3** secondary to the carcinoma **2** .

Remember Pancoast's tumour – bronchogenic carcinoma in the apex of the lung associated with Horner's syndrome (unilateral ptosis, miosis, enophthalmos and hyperhydrosis).

Investigation
A chest radiograph (Fig. 3.10) is commonly used to detect broncho-genic carcinoma **2** , which may be radiologically staged using CT or MRI scanning. Sputum cytology, broncho-scopic washings, brushings or biopsy may be used to establish the histo-logical diagnosis.

Treatment
Surgical resection is rarely possible but offers the prospect of cure for early stage lesions. Combination chemotherapy or chemoradiotherapy and symptom relief are the mainstays of palliative treatment.

Table 3.3 Features of right bronchial carcinoma		
	Right	**Left**
Chest expansion	Reduced	Normal
Percussion note	Dull over affected part of lung	Normal
Breath sounds	Bronchial over affected part of lung	Normal
Added sounds	Crepitations + rhonchi over affected part of lung	Normal
Vocal resonance	May be increased over affected part of lung	Normal

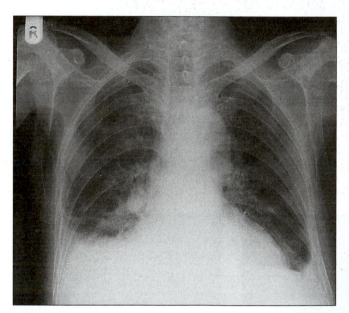

Fig. 3.10 Bronchial carcinoma

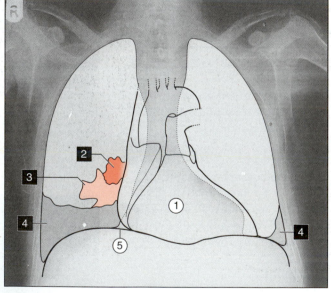

KEY

① Heart
② Bronchogenic carcinoma
③ Consolidation and lung collapse
④ Bilateral pleural effusion
⑤ Diaphragm

Pleural effusion

History
Pleural effusion is usually secondary to diseases in other organs. Hence, pay particular attention to cardiac and respiratory symptoms and treatments, and past medical history including intra-abdominal surgery or conditions such as pancreatitis and malignancy (particularly lung, breast and GI).

Examination (Table 3.4)
On **inspection**, look for cachexia, increased respiratory rate and signs of vomiting (thinking of aspiration).

On **palpation**, look for diminished chest expansion on the affected side and reduced or absent vocal resonance.

On **percussion**, listen for a stony dull note over the effusion (Fig. 3.11 **2**), but resonance above the effusion over normal lung. Remember the position of the liver and that pleural effusions may be bilateral **2** .

On **auscultation**, listen for absence of breath sounds over effusion, sometimes with bronchial breathing at the top of effusion and normal breath sounds superiorly.

Investigation
A PA chest radiograph (Fig. 3.11) which may be supplemented by a lateral view (Fig. 3.12) demonstrates loss of the costophrenic angle. Aspiration of the effusion (following localization of the dull area by either percussion or ultrasound) enables cytological, bacteriological and biochemical analysis.

Exudate (protein >30 g/l) may be due to:
- primary or secondary malignancy
- infection
- intra-abdominal inflammation (pancreatitis)
- sepsis (subphrenic abscess).

A transudate (protein <30 g/l) suggests a medical cause (heart failure, cirrhosis, nephrotic syndrome).

Treatment
Drainage of the effusion and treatment of the underlying cause.

Table 3.4 Features of right pleural effusion

	Right	Left
Chest expansion	Reduced	Normal
Percussion note	Stony dull	Normal
Breath sounds	Absent or decreased (occasionally bronchial)	Normal
Added sounds	None	Normal
Vocal resonance	Absent or decreased	Normal

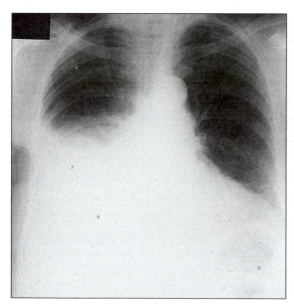
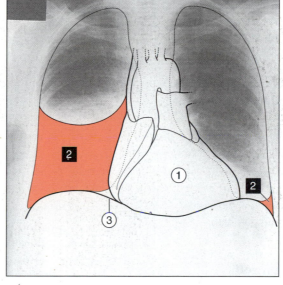

KEY
① Heart
2 Pleural effusion
③ Diaphragm

Fig. 3.11 Pleural effusion

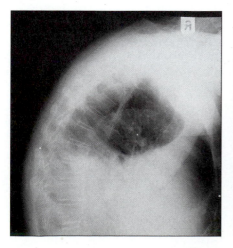
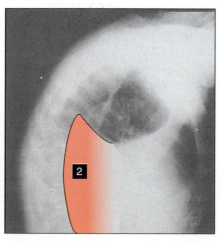

Fig. 3.12 Lateral chest radiograph of pleaural effusion

Heart disorders

Cardiac surgery may be performed as an open procedure through a midline sternotomy or thoracotomy or, increasingly, via transarterial (usually femoral) routes (angioplasty, stenting) or minimally invasive endoscopic techniques. Coronary artery disease, secondary to atheroma, and valve disease, secondary to rheumatic fever, infective endocarditis or congenital valve disease, are the common reasons for surgical intervention in cardiac surgery. The aortic and mitral valves are the two most commonly replaced valves in surgical practice.

It is useful to know why cardio-vascular disease is of importance in surgical practice. A history of angina, hypertension, myocardial infarction or aortic stenosis places the patient at increased risk of a further cardiac event or even death in surgical practice. Surgical intervention within 6 months of a myocardial infarction, and particularly within 6 weeks, places the patient at high risk of a further, potentially fatal, myocardial infarction. In addition, the American Society of Anesthesiologists' (ASA) grading system indicates, on the basis of the severity of pre-existing disease (often cardiorespiratory), a patient's risk of death as a result of surgery.

ASA grading
ASA 1 – normal
ASA 2 – mild/moderate systemic
      disturbance
ASA 3 – severe systemic disturbance
ASA 4 – life-threatening systemic
      disorder
ASA 5 – moribund patient with little
      chance of survival.

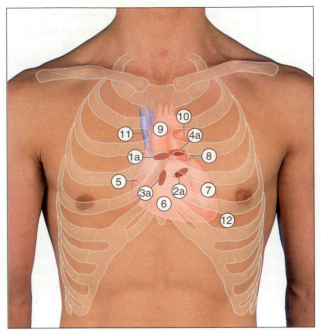

Fig. 3.13a Cardiac anatomy in relation to the chest wall

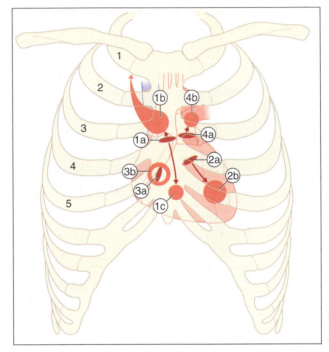

Fig. 3.13b Position of heart valves and sites for auscultation

KEY

① Aortic valve
① Aortic stenosis murmur area
① Aortic regurgitation murmur area
② Mitral valve
② Mitral murmur area
③ Tricuspid valve
③ Tricuspid murmur area
④ Pulmonary valve
④ Pulmonary stenosis murmur area

⑤ Right atrium
⑥ Right ventricle
⑦ Left ventricle
⑧ Left atrial appendage
⑨ Aorta
⑩ Pulmonary artery
⑪ Superior vena cava
⑫ 5th intercostal space (apex beat)

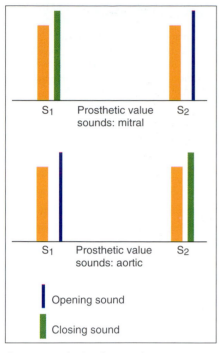

Fig. 3.14 Prosthetic valve sounds

History
The patient's age will suggest the likely underlying pathology. Congenital and infective problems are more common in young people. A full cardiovascular history should include current and past symptoms of chest pain (on exercise or at rest, whether relieved by glyceryle trinitrate (GTN)), breathlessness (on exercise, at rest, when lying flat), intermittent claudication (which part(s) of the limbs and distance before claudication occurs) and whether this is stable or progressive. A past history of myocardial infarction, transient ischaemic attack or stroke, diabetes (insulin-dependent or diet/drug controlled), rheumatic fever, hypertension, a current history of medications and a family history are all required. In a young person, ask about congenital heart disease – have problems been present since childhood? Information should be obtained about foreign travel, drug addiction (thinking of infective endocarditis with valve destruction) and foreign travel or animal contacts for more exotic infective agents (such as Q fever).

Many patients are aware of the results of previous investigations or procedures such as echocardiography (ultrasound of the heart valves and myocardium for structure and function), coronary or cardiac angiography (performed through femoral puncture), radionuclide scans for cardiac function or insertion of a pacemaker.

Most patients who have had one or more valves replaced know the type of valve and the medical implications such as anticoagulation for mechanical valves and antibacterial prophylaxis for all invasive procedures including dental work, regardless of the type of valve.

Examination
On **inspection**, look for signs of cardiac disease: increased respiratory rate, central cyanosis, peripheral oedema, bruising from anticoagulant therapy and surgical scars. With the patient at 45 degrees, measure the jugulovenous pressure. Listen for the tell-tale click of heart valves.

On **palpation**, starting with the hands, look for finger clubbing (Fig. 3.2) (congenital heart disease), palmar erythema (mitral valve disease), Roth spots or splinter haemorrhage (infective endocarditis).

Feel for the radial pulse for rate, rhythm (regular, irregular), force and character (collapsing or normal in nature); palpate for radiofemoral delay (coarctation of the aorta).

Check the blood pressure, remembering to use an adequately sized and correctly positioned cuff. Palpate for the apex beat (which should be in the fifth intercostal space in the midclavicular line; Fig. 3.13a ⑫, Table 3.5) and for thrills and heaves (Table 3.6).

Table 3.5 Abnormalities of the apex beat	
Diffuse or dyskinetic	Post-infarction; left ventricular aneurysm
Sustained or 'heaving'	Left ventricular hypertrophy
Double impulse	Hypertrophic cardiomyopathy
Hyperkinetic	Mitral reflux: shunts

Table 3.6 Lesions which cause thrills	
Systolic thrills	**Diastolic thrills**
Aortic stenosis	Mitral stenosis
Ventricular septal defect	Tricuspid stenosis
Pulmonary stenosis	

On **auscultation**, listen for murmurs over the apex and anterior chest with the diaphragm of the stethoscope (Fig. 3.13b). The bell is useful for listening for low pitched sounds, the diaphragm for high pitched sounds. Listen for a pericardial rub and for cardiac murmurs (Table 3.7). The radiation of murmurs is in the direction of blood flow (Fig. 3.13b). The common murmurs radiate to the neck (aortic stenosis, Fig. 3.13 (1b)), to the parasternal region with the patient sitting forward (aortic regurgitation (1c)), and towards the axilla with the patient rolled on one side (listen with the bell, mitral regurgitation (2b)). Clearly, cardiac murmurs in a patient who has not had surgery will be very different after surgery has been performed. Following surgery, the opening and or closing click of the valves and any associated flow murmurs will precisely coincide with diastole or systole, depending on which valve or valves have been replaced (Fig. 3.14).

Investigation

Investigation of patients with cardiac disease can be extensive. In addition to routine haematology and biochemistry, biochemical tests include blood glucose and indicators of diabetic control if the patient is diabetic, lipids and cholesterol, and thyroid status; haematological tests include anticoagulant status (by international normalized ratio for patients receiving warfarin). Further investigation will include chest radiology (PA and lateral). Echocardiography can be used to examine the structure and function of the heart muscle, heart valves and blood flow. Radionuclide techniques and invasive techniques such as angiography can be used to assess coronary arteries, cardiac valves and cardiac muscle function.

Treatment of valve disease sometimes (though not exclusively) requires replacement of one or more valves (Fig. 3.15) **4**. Treatment of dysrhythmia may merit placement of a pacemaker **3**.

Table 3.7 Cardiac murmurs	
Condition	**Type of murmur**
Aortic stenosis	Ejection systolic murmur Radiates to carotids
Aortic regurgitation	Early diastolic murmur Left sternal edge Best heard with the patient leaning forward, on expiration
Mitral stenosis	Mid-diastolic murmur At apex
Mitral regurgitation	Pansystolic murmur At apex Radiates to axilla Best heard with the patient in the left lateral position, using the bell of the stethoscope

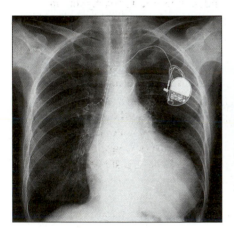
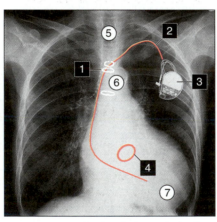

KEY

1	Sternal wire
2	Pacing wire
3	Pacemaker
4	Aortic valve replacement
(5)	Trachea
(6)	Aorta
(7)	Left ventricle

Fig. 3.15 Chest radiograph of pacemaker

4 Breast

Breast symptoms (breast lumps, breast pain, nipple discharge) are common in the female population. While 1 in 12 women in the UK develop breast cancer during their lifetime, only 1 in 10 women attending a hospital breast clinic will have breast cancer. This chapter outlines how to take a history and examine a woman with breast symptoms and illustrates common clinical processes.

The breast sits upon the muscles of the chest wall (Fig. 4.1 ① ⑧) and has important relationships to the axillary contents ④ ⑤ ⑥ ⑦.

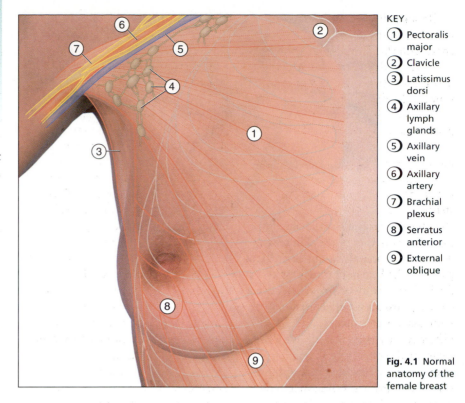

KEY
① Pectoralis major
② Clavicle
③ Latissimus dorsi
④ Axillary lymph glands
⑤ Axillary vein
⑥ Axillary artery
⑦ Brachial plexus
⑧ Serratus anterior
⑨ External oblique

Fig. 4.1 Normal anatomy of the female breast

History
The history should include questions related to the specific breast complaint on each side.

Lump. When was it first noted? How has it changed since then? What is its position, shape, mobility and is it tender? Is there any cyclical variation (e.g. increase in size before menses, decrease after menses)?

Skin changes. These include redness, swelling, peau d'orange (orange skin) appearance, eczema of the nipple (especially if unilateral and no eczema elsewhere, when there is a need to exclude Paget's disease, intradermal cancer, of the nipple).

Nipple retraction. If unilateral, asymmetrical and distorting, it may be due to an underlying cancer.

Nipple discharge. Ask if single or multiple, what colour it is, and whether blood stained (single duct blood stained nipple discharge may be due to duct papilloma or carcinoma) or galactorrhoea.

Pain. Are changes cyclical or acyclical (i.e. no changes with menses)? Is pain unilateral or unifocal.

Other relevant history:
- Age (Fig. 4.2)
- Menopausal status
- Menstrual history
- Hormonal medications
- Gynaecological history
- Family history of breast cancer.
  General health questions:
- Past medical history of medical conditions
- Surgical operations
- Medications
- Allergies
- Smoking (associated with inflammatory processes in the breast)
- Symptoms suggestive of metastatic disease: breathlessness, musculoskeletal aches, tiredness, anorexia.

Breast examination
Exposure. With a chaperone present (particularly if you are male), ask the woman for permission to examine her and request she removes her clothing from the upper half of her body.

Inspection (Fig. 4.3 a, b, c). Note that the size, shape and ptosis of the breast vary markedly between individuals and for each woman change with the monthly cycle, with pregnancy and with age.

With the woman sitting, naked to waist (Fig. 4.3a), ask her to raise her arms above her head and lean forward (Fig. 4.3b), then with her hands on her hips to tense the pectoral muscles (Fig. 4.3c). These actions accentuate skin contour or dimpling changes due to underlying breast pathology.

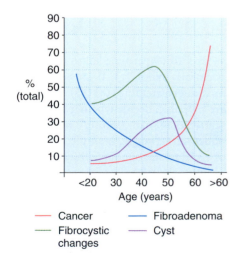

Fig. 4.2 Some types of breast lump are more common at certain ages as a percentage of all lumps at that age

— Cancer
— Fibrocystic changes
— Fibroadenoma
— Cyst

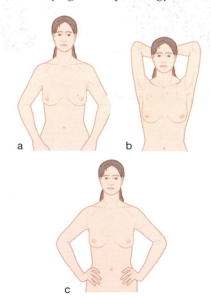

Fig. 4.3 Patient positioning for inspection of changes in breast pathology

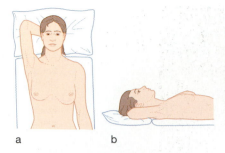

Fig. 4.4 Position of the patient for right breast examination.

Look for surgical scars (which may be difficult to spot in the skin creases or around the nipple), signs of previous radiotherapy (telangiectasia, skin tattoo, thin, shiny or thickened coarse skin) or the encrusted eczematous nipple of Paget's disease.

Palpation (Fig. 4.4a, b). With the patient as comfortable as possible, lying flat on a couch or bed with one pillow, examine each breast systematically in turn. First ask the patient where any tender areas are (examine these areas last of all and be particularly gentle there) and ask her to point to any specific lumps.

Examine the normal side first; ask the patient to place her hand behind her head on the side being examined (Fig. 4.4a).

Use gentle palpation with flattened fingers compressing the breast tissue against the chest wall and a rotating movement. Move around the breast, initially palpating superficially then deeper, to examine all four quadrants of the breast and the axillary tail.

Remember to be particularly careful with the tender breast and also examine behind the nipple/areolar regions. If the history has suggested a nipple discharge, ask the patient to squeeze the breast to produce discharge (and use a urinary dipstick to test for blood).

Where a lump is detected, describe its side, position (as if on a clock face) and shape. Measure its size (using

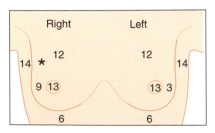

Fig. 4.5 Record the findings using positions of the clock (13 = central, 14 = axillary tail)

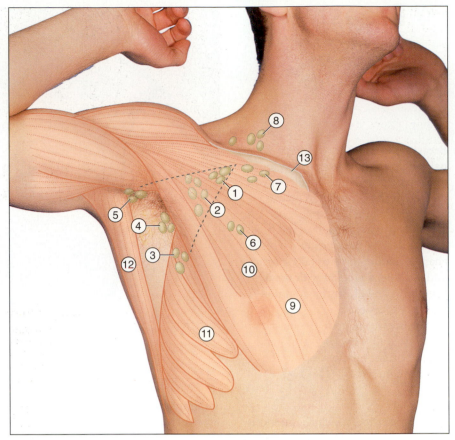

Fig. 4.6 Normal anatomy of the axilla and lymph nodes

KEY

① Apical (level III) lymph nodes
② Level II nodes posterior to pectoralis minor
③ Medial ⎫
④ Posterior ⎬ level I nodes
⑤ Lateral ⎭
⑥ Interpectoral nodes – between pectoralis major and minor
⑦ Infraclavicular nodes
⑧ Supraclavicular nodes
⑨ Pectoralis major
⑩ Pectoralis minor
⑪ Serratus anterior
⑫ Latissimus dorsi
⑬ Clavicle

calipers). Check mobility of the lump, any tethering to skin, tethering or fixity to pectoralis major or chest wall, and its consistency: hard, craggy, soft, tender, fluctuant. Record your findings on a diagram (Fig. 4.5).

Axillary examination

Although clinical examination of lymph nodes, particularly in the axilla, is a poor marker for nodal involvement in breast cancer, regional node examination of the axillary (Fig. 4.6 ①–⑤), infraclavicular ⑦, supraclavicular ⑧, and cervical nodes completes clinical examination of the breast. Axillary examination may also be required in men when looking for generalized lymphadenopathy.

Examine both sides, starting with the presumed normal side. To examine the right side, with the patient lying on their back or sitting, rest their right forearm on your right forearm and use your left hand to gently examine the four walls of the axilla – medial, posterior, lateral and anterior – taking care to feel right up into the apex of the axilla (Fig. 4.6 ①). The position of axillary nodes is described in relation to the pectoralis minor muscle

as level III (supero-medial to the pectoralis minor, ①) II (posterior ②) or I (inferolateral ③ ④ ⑤). If nodes are palpable, decide whether they are scattered 4–8mm ('shotty') normal nodes, large, single, multiple, matted or fixed to surrounding structures. To examine the left side, take the patient's left forearm in your left hand and examine their left axilla with your right hand.

Examination of the clavicular fossae and the neck is often most comfortably accomplished (for both you and the patient) by standing behind the patient, who should be seated (see Ch. 2).

Investigations

Clinical, radiological and cyto/pathological assessment are used to determine whether a breast lesion is benign or malignant (Fig. 4.8). This is called triple assessment.

Radiological assessment. Mammograms (Fig. 4.7) are used to detect distortions in architecture, masses **2** and/or micro-calcification and are more effective in the over-35-years age group, as the density of breast tissue generally declines with age. Breast ultrasound is particularly useful in younger women and should differentiate between a benign lump, a cyst and a cancer. Breast screening (in the UK) uses mammography every 3 years between the ages of 50 and 70 and aims to detect early cancers or precancerous lesions.

Cytological and pathological assessment. Fine needle aspiration cytology (FNAC) involves passing a fine needle (e.g. 19G) into, and aspiration from, the area of tissue to be sampled. A cytopathologist can then examine the stained slides for the cytological features of benign, atypical or malignant cells. Core biopsy (using a larger needle under anaesthesia) or open biopsy may be used to establish the diagnosis.

Other investigations. The following investigations may also be appropriate in the diagnosis and staging of breast and axillary abnormalities:

- full blood count (for anaemia, marrow infiltration, or before and after chemotherapy), ESR/plasma viscosity
- blood biochemistry (urea, electrolytes, creatinine and liver function tests)
- chest radiograph (PA) for metastases, static isotope bone scan and liver ultrasound scan to stage larger cancers or where metastatic disease is suspected.

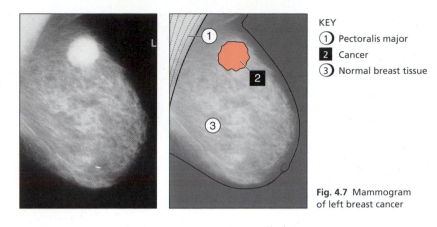

KEY
(1) Pectoralis major
2 Cancer
(3) Normal breast tissue

Fig. 4.7 Mammogram of left breast cancer

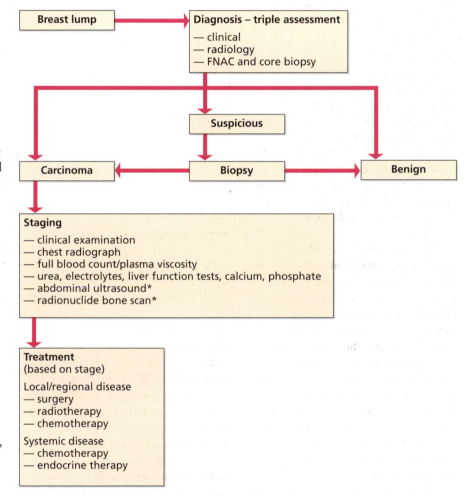

Fig. 4.8 Management of a breast lump (*in more advanced disease)

Breast cancer

History

A new breast lump in a woman over 35 years should be considered to be a breast cancer until proven otherwise. Ask about the features of the lump, skin changes, nipple changes (see Figs 4.10 and 4.11 **6** – **9**); breast-related changes, especially menopausal status (which influences choice of therapy), and hormonal medications.

The past history of breast conditions should include details of previous surgery and, if a cancer has been previously treated, how (surgery, radiotherapy, endocrine or chemotherapy).

General health questions should include those outlined on page 25.

Examination

Ask permission to examine the patient, then perform a systematic inspection and palpation of both breasts (Figs. 4.3, 4.4) and the regional lymph nodes (Fig. 4.6). Figure 4.9 shows the normal female anatomy.

Examine any other symptomatic tissues, e.g. the musculoskeletal system for bone metastases, the liver for metastatic disease.

Investigations

Investigation of a breast lump is on the basis of 'triple assessment', that is, clinical assessment (history and examination findings), radiological assessment (two-view mammography supplemented by breast ultrasound, or in the under 35 age group ultrasound alone) and cytology/pathology assessment (fine needle aspiration cytology or, under anaesthetic, core needle biopsy or open surgical biopsy. Triple assessment will establish or refute the diagnosis of breast cancer. Following diagnosis, the cancer is staged to assess the extent of the disease using the TNM system (see Table 4.1) and treatment options offered to the patient according to the stage of the disease and her general health.

The patient in Figure 4.10 presented with a palpable breast lump. Note the

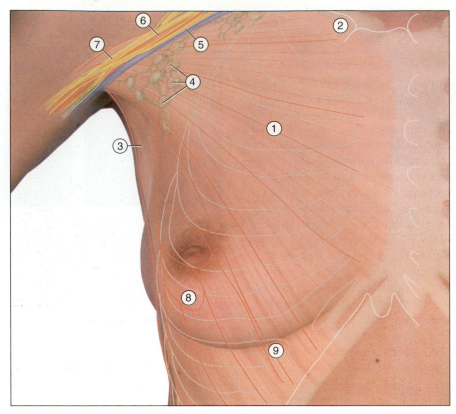

Fig. 4.9 Normal anatomy of the female chest

KEY
1. Pectoralis major
2. Clavicle
3. Latissimus dorsi
4. Axillary lymph glands
5. Axillary vein
6. Axillary artery
7. Brachial plexus
8. Serratus anterior
9. External oblique

skin tethering **7** as the woman raises her arm and the nipple retraction **6** .

The patient in Figure 4.11 presented with indrawn nipple **6** and skin tethering **7** with skin involvement by the cancer **9** . Note also palpable axillary lymph glands **10** .

Treatment

Surgery. Either lumpectomy (small cancer in large breast) or mastectomy (where the cancer is large relative to breast size, or multi-focal, or by patient choice) may be performed.

Surgery to the axilla involves

Table 4.1 Staging of breast cancer		
Tumours	T	cancer clinically <2 cm
	T2	cancer clinically 2–5 cm
	T3	cancer clinically >5 cm
	T4	cancer involving skin or chest wall.
Nodes	N0	no regional node metastasis
	N1	metatasis to movable ipsilateral axillary nodes
	N2	metatasis to fixed ipsilateral axillary nodes
Metastasis	M0	no metastasis
	M1	distant metastasis

clearance or selective removal of nodes (node sample or sentinel node biopsy).

Radiotherapy. Treatment is given to breast/chest wall and metastases.

Chemotherapy. Systemic treatment is 'adjuvant' in women at risk of future recurrent disease, or 'therapeutic' to treat advanced disease in the breast or metastatic spread.

Endocrine therapy. Antihormonal treatment is particularly effective in women who have had hormone receptor-bearing cancers (e.g. tamoxifen tablets in postmenopausal women).

Complications of breast surgery and breast cancer surgery
Local
- Bleeding
- Haematoma
- Infection
- Seroma
- Nerve damage (or loss of abnormal sensation)
- Lymphoedema

General
- Atelectasis,
- Chest infection
- DVT/PE

KEY
1. Clavicle
2. Pectoralis major
3. Pectoralis minor
4. Latissimus dorsi
5. Areola
6. Indrawn nipple
7. Skin tethering
8. Site of cancer
9. Cancer infiltrating skin
10. Node mass

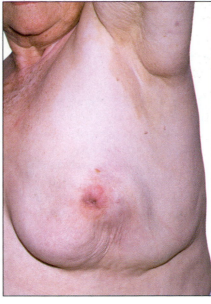
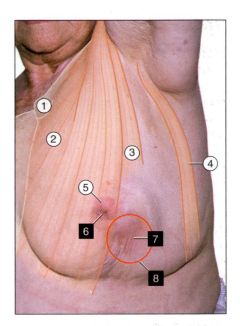

Fig. 4.10 Palpable breast lump

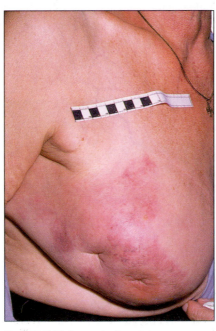
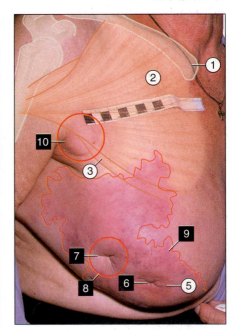

Fig. 4.11 Withdrawn nipple

Fibroadenoma and breast cyst

A fibroadenoma (Fig. 4.12) is considered an aberration of normal development and involution (ANDI). It typically occurs in a woman under 30 years of age. A breast cyst (Fig. 4.13) typically occurs in women aged 35–55 years.

History

Age is important (review Fig. 4.2). Ask about the features of the lump – particularly any change in size, tenderness and the presence of more than one. Include a full breast and general history.

A fibroadenoma (Fig. 4.12 **7**) is usually very mobile, discrete, rounded, 1–2 cm in size, and does not change with a woman's menses. There may be more than one. Cysts may be single (Fig. 4.13 **8**) or multiple, unilateral or bilateral, and range in size from a few mm to several cm.

Examination

Inspection may reveal the site of the lump if it lies superficially (Fig. 4.12 **7**, Fig. 4.13 **8**). Having first examined the normal breast, ask the patient to locate the lump. Then examine the affected breast, arriving finally at the lump to exclude any other breast abnormalities.

With a fibroadenoma (Fig. 4.12 **7**), confirm the position, smooth outline, mobile firm lump and record the size with calipers. A cyst is often smooth in outline (Fig. 4.13 **8**) and can be variable in size.

Investigations and treatment

All breast lumps require triple assessment. Clinical assessment is followed by mammography and/or breast ultrasound (if the patient is less than 35 years old) then fine needle aspiration cytology (FNAC).

If these findings confirm the diagnosis of a fibroadenoma (Fig. 4.12 **7**), either excisional biopsy is performed or the lump is re-examined after 6–12 months (no change in size or regression means it can be safely left alone).

With a cyst (Fig. 4.13 **8**), aspiration can be both diagnostic and therapeutic. The cyst fluid may be clear, yellow, green or even very dark. Frank blood in the aspirate or a residual mass (which should have a separate FNA) may signal the presence of a cancer within the wall of the cyst. Cysts may recur either at the same site or elsewhere in the breast.

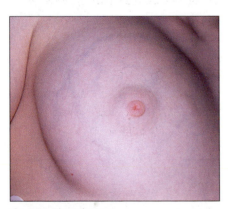
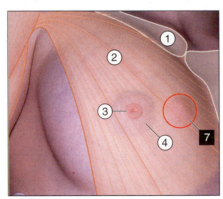

KEY
1. Clavicle
2. Pectoralis major
3. Nipple
4. Areola
5. Pectoralis minor
6. Latissimus dorsi
7 Fibroadenoma
8 Breast cyst

Fig. 4.12 Fibroadenoma

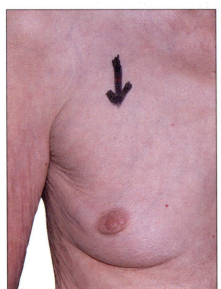
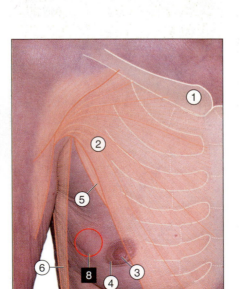

  Fig. 4.13 Breast cyst

Axillary mass

Axillary lumps may occur in men or women of all ages, but are commonly regional lymphadenopathy (review Figs 4.1 and 4.6) associated with local abnormalities in the breast (particularly breast cancer) or lymphadenopathy from systemic diseases (commonly viral infections). The neurovascular structures in the axilla, particularly the axillary vein (Fig. 4.14 ①), neurovascular bundle to latissimus dorsi ⑥, long thoracic nerve to serratus anterior ⑦ and intercostobrachial nerve ③ are vulnerable to surgical damage when removing axillary nodes.

History

The history should include the patient's age and the features of the axillary lump or lumps (Fig. 4.15 **4**): when first noted, size, change in size, shape, whether single or multiple, unilateral or bilateral, the position, mobility, tenderness, any cyclical variation (e.g. increase in size before menses, decrease after menses), and any skin changes over the lump.

Associated features should include any restriction of upper limb movements, any swelling of the upper limb (see Fig. 4.17), or symptoms of systemic upset.

Examination

Following inspection for any obvious axillary lumps (Fig. 4.15 **4**), examin-ation of the axilla concentrates on palpating the medial (chest wall), posterior (subscapularis, latissimus dorsi), lateral (humeral) and anterior (pectoralis major and minor) walls of the axilla and palpating into the apical region. Palpation should compare the right and left sides and then go on to examine the infraclavicular, supra-clavicular and cervical regions (Ch. 2) for additional lymphadenopathy. The breasts should be examined (see pp. 25–26) to exclude a primary breast source for the axillary lump.

Investigation

For a localized axillary mass, fine needle aspiration cytology may provide the diagnosis. If axillary lymphaden-opathy is part of generalized lymph-adenopathy then investigations suggested in Chapter 2 (p. 9) may be appropriate.

Treatment

Excisional biopsy may both remove the lump and provide a definitive diagnosis.

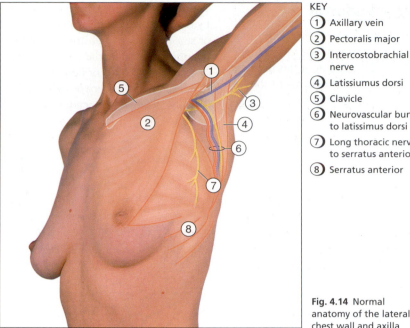

KEY
① Axillary vein
② Pectoralis major
③ Intercostobrachial nerve
④ Latissiumus dorsi
⑤ Clavicle
⑥ Neurovascular bundle to latissimus dorsi
⑦ Long thoracic nerve to serratus anterior
⑧ Serratus anterior

Fig. 4.14 Normal anatomy of the lateral chest wall and axilla

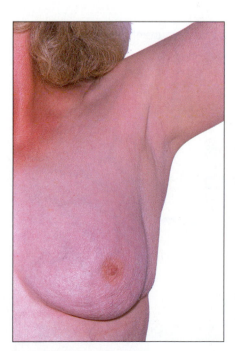

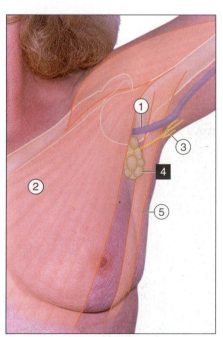

KEY
① Axillary vein
② Pectoralis major
③ Intercostobrachial nerve (T2)
4 Axillary lump (mass of nodes)
⑤ Latissimus dorsi

Fig. 4.15 Palpable axillary lump

Lymphoedema

The upper limb and breast depend on the axillary lymph nodes for drainage (Fig. 4.16). Disruption of this drainage may result in lymphoedema of the arm and breast on that side.

History

Ask about the onset, duration and severity of the upper limb swelling. Did it start after injury, infection or therapy (axillary surgery or axillary radiotherapy in particular)? Has it worsened since first noted? Does the swelling affect the fingers (are rings tight?), hand, wrist, forearm, upper arm; is there difficulty bending digits, the wrist or elbow? Does clothing still fit or does the swelling cause embarrassment and need to be covered up? Has the patient tried any measures to reduce the swelling (arm elevation, massage, compression armlet)?

Examination

On inspection, look at the relative distribution of the swelling (Fig. 4.17) and compare the right and left sides. Are rings, a wrist watch or clothing tight **4** ? Can the patient fully flex the digits, wrist and elbow joints? Inspect the axillary region, trunk (anterior and posterior), clavicular and cervical regions for surgical scars, signs of radiotherapy, skin changes **2** , **9** , lumps or swellings. Palpate the axillary contents as outlined above, seeking a cause for the upper limb swelling. Continue on to examine the neck and chest wall for palpable abnormalities **2** **5** **6** **9** .

Investigation

Investigation should aim to determine the cause of the lymphoedema. This may be clinically obvious (Fig. 4.17) or require radiological assessment for which MRI provides good detail.

KEY
1. Clavicle
2. Cancer infiltrating skin and lymphatics
3. Pectoralis major
4. Compression mark from arm stocking
5. Areola
6. Nipple
7. Arm stocking wound down
8. Lymphoedematous arm
9. Cancer infiltrating skin of breast

Treatment

Lymphoedema may be primary (rare) or secondary due to obstruction of the lymphatics draining the upper limb by cancer (Fig 4.17 **2**) or destruction of the drainage by surgery or radiotherapy. Treatment depends on the cause but is often aimed at mechanically reducing the swelling by elevation of the limb, massage or mechanical compression ⑦. Therapy for carcinoma causing obstruction may also be worthwhile.

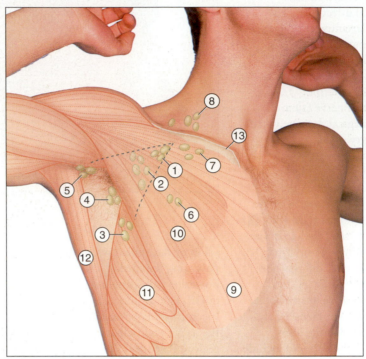

Fig. 4.16 Normal anatomy of the axilla and lymph nodes

KEY
① Apical (level III) lymph nodes
② Level II nodes posterior to pectoralis minor
③ Medial ⎫
④ Posterior ⎬ level I nodes
⑤ Lateral ⎭
⑥ Interpectoral nodes – between pectoralis major and minor
⑦ Infraclavicular nodes
⑧ Supraclavicular nodes
⑨ Pectoralis major
⑩ Pectoralis minor
⑪ Serratus anterior
⑫ Latissimus dorsi
⑬ Clavicle

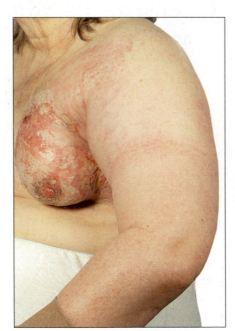
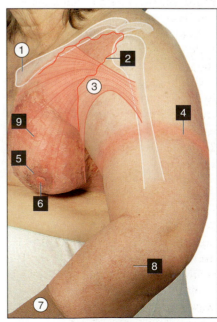

Fig. 4.17 Lymphoedema of upper limb secondary to advanced breast cancer

5 Abdomen

The abdominal contents lie hidden behind a sometimes substantial abdominal wall, the localization of pain may be poor and several structures lie close to each other (Figs 5.1 and 5.2); knowledge of the abdominal anatomy is therefore actually useful in clinical practice. The patient's history supplemented by clinical examination and investigation should identify the underlying problem.

History

Some important general questions often get overlooked in considering the abdomen, but may point to the diagnosis. These include the age, gender, occupation, social history (alcohol intake, smoking), and drug history (as a potential cause of abdominal symptoms, or taken to relieve abdominal symptoms). Family history may be important for a range of abdominal problems including colon cancer and inflammatory bowel disease.

Systemic manifestations of abdominal disease processes include loss of appetite, weight loss or weight gain (in kg or lb, or measured by change in size of clothing or belt), nausea, pallor, jaundice, itch and bruising.

Systematic questions about the abdominal gastrointestinal tract should include:

Swallowing. If there is difficulty swallowing, ask about onset, duration, and any progression from solids (often meat is the first problem noted) to liquids or even inability to swallow saliva.

Vomiting. What is its timing in relation to food ingestion? Is the food recognizable or partly/fully digested? What is the colour of the vomitus – opalescent fluid (pure gastric juice), brown (bile), green (proximal small bowel), faeculent (distal small bowel)?

Waterbrash. Ask if there is regurgitation of gastric contents into the oesophagus and pharynx.

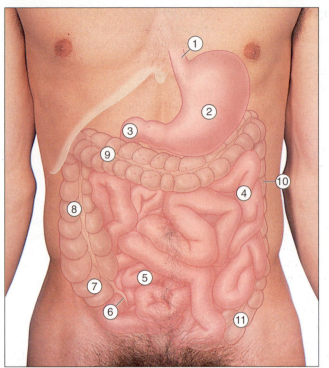

KEY
1. Oesophagus
2. Stomach
3. Duodenum
4. Jejunum
5. Ileum
6. Appendix
7. Caecum
8. Ascending colon
9. Transverse colon
10. Descending colon
11. Sigmoid colon

Fig. 5.1 Surface markings of the alimentary tract

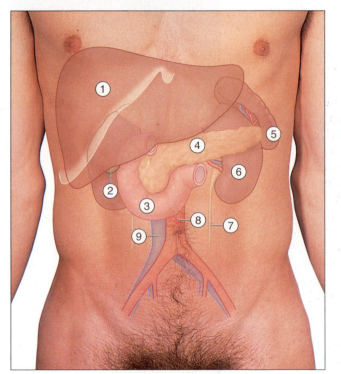

KEY
1. Liver
2. Gall bladder
3. Duodenum
4. Pancreas
5. Spleen
6. Kidney
7. Ureter
8. Aorta
9. Vena cava

Fig. 5.2 Surface markings of the abdominal viscera

Indigestion or heartburn. Ask if there is a burning sensation in the epigastrium.

Abdominal pain. This can be described in detail by a patient in response to the following questions and strongly suggests the likely diagnosis.
- When did the pain start?
- Where does it occur?
- When does it occur?
- Can the pain be described (sharp/dull/burning/gripping)?
- How often does the pain occur (periodicity)?
- Where does the pain radiate to?
- What are the aggravating factors?
- What are the relieving factors?
- What are the associated features?

Abdominal distension (bloating). If this occurs, is it intermittent (and what is the periodicity) or progressive? When was the first episode and how often does it occur?

Bowel habit. Has there been any change in bowel habit, increasing constipation or diarrhoea, either of which may be intermittent or progressive?

What are the consistency, colour, smell and features of the stool, and how has the stool changed recently? Does the stool flush away easily or with difficulty?

Has the patient noted any blood, mucus or pus passed per anum? If blood was noted was it fresh red blood or old dark blood, clots or liquid, mixed in with the stool or separate from the stool or on the toilet paper only? Did this occur once or on multiple occasions?

Is there any pain on defaecation or any faecal or urinary incontinence? Have there been problems with itch, abscesses or fistulae in the area?

Gynaecological history. This should include the date of the last menstrual period, whether the patient is currently pregnant, the number of pregnancies and mode of delivery. Ask whether there is vaginal discharge, midcycle pain, pain at the time of menses, or intermenstrual or post-menopausal bleeding.

Past medical history. The past medical history should include previous surgery and medical illnesses, and past drug use (prescribed and 'recreational'). History of jaundice, travel abroad, contact with farm or household animals and sexual history, may all be of relevance to abdominal diagnoses.

Examination

Abdominal examination may be facilitated by first examining other parts of the body (hands, head and neck, lower limbs) for systemic signs of intra-abdominal conditions. Look for the following:

- hands: finger clubbing (Fig. 3.2), palmar erythema, Dupuytren's contracture, leuconychia
- head and neck: jaundice of the sclera (Fig. 5.3) or pallor of the conjunctiva, spider naevi, telangiectasia, perioral pigmented spots
- chest: gynaecomastia, missing breast (Fig. 5.5 **2**) (for intra-abdominal metastases from breast cancer)
- lower limbs: peripheral oedema, scratch marks, bruising, erythema nodosum.

Exposure/positioning. Position the patient lying comfortably flat on his back, head resting on one pillow, and exposed from nipple to groin so that you can see and subsequently feel the abdomen.

Inspection. Close inspection can give you many clues as to what you may find during subsequent palpation, percussion and auscultation. Watch for movement (or lack of movement due to abdominal pain) on respiration, visible peristalsis, abdominal masses or asymmetry.

Look for surgical scars (Fig. 5.4), not only on the anterior abdominal wall but in the flanks, in the groin (perhaps hidden by hair or fat), at the umbilicus and on the chest wall. Small surgical scars (from laparoscopy) and skin crease incisions can heal remarkably well.

Look for obvious features such as a stoma (Fig. 5.55, p.60) which may be hidden by a stoma bag, fistulae, masses, and skin changes (distended veins, skin lesions, bruising, erythema ab igne, Fig. 5.10).

If an abdominal mass is apparent, ask the patient to raise his head off the pillow to try to determine whether the mass is intra-abdominal (the mass disappears) or on the surface of the abdominal wall (the mass persists). Ask the patient to give a big cough to emphasize any hernias (e.g. incisional hernia secondary to previous surgery, Fig. 7.3) and look to see if the patient winces because of abdominal pain when coughing or moving.

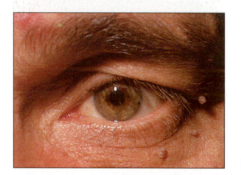

Fig. 5.3 Jaundice of sclera

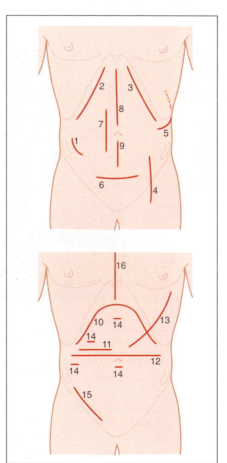

Fig. 5.4 Abdominal scars

KEY

1   Lanz (appendix)
2   Kocher's (hepatobiliary)
3   Left subcostal (spleen)
4   Vascular
5   Nephrectomy (extraperitoneal)
6   Pfannenstiel (gynaecology or caesarean section)
7   Right paramedian
8   Upper midline
9   Lower midline
10   Roof-top (pancreatobiliary)
11   Transverse (gall bladder, colectomy)
12   Transverse (abdominal aortic aneurysm, colonic surgery)
13   Thoracoabdominal (extending over left thorax; gastro-oesophageal surgery)
14   Laparoscopic port sites (for laparoscopic cholecystectomy)
15   Inguinal hernia
16   Sternotomy

Palpation. Ask the patient's permission to palpate the abdomen and ask where the abdomen is sorest so that you can avoid touching that area until last. Kneeling beside the patient, on the patient's right hand side, watch the patient's face (to see if you are causing discomfort) and, using the flat of your hand, gently palpate the four quadrants of the abdomen. Follow this superficial palpation with deeper palpation to locate and delineate abdominal masses. If you can feel a mass, define the boundaries and extent of the mass where you can: What is the position and the size of the mass? Is it mobile? Is it possible to indent the mass (e.g. faeces palpable in the colon)? Is it expansile (aortic aneurysm)? Is the mass ballottable (kidney)?

Rectal examination using a gloved and lubricated finger will allow you to describe the sphincter tone, palpate the prostate in males (size, smooth/craggy, whether tender), and palpate the cervix in females (whether tender). Feel the rectal mucosa for any abnormalities and obtain a sample of faeces for occult blood testing.

Vaginal examination using two gloved lubricated fingers may be appropriate to palpate the gynaecological organs.

Percussion. Percussion is useful to distinguish hollow structures from solid structures and to define their borders. Gentle percussion of the acute abdomen is a much kinder way to elicit rebound than the traditional sudden release of deep palpation. Percussion to seek shifting dullness (Fig. 5.5) detects the boundary between dull ▮1 and resonant ③ percussion notes in the abdomen; the patient then rolls over and, if shifting dullness is present (and thus ascites), the dull percussion note becomes resonant as the air-filled intestine ③ floats on top of the fluid.

Auscultation. Using the diaphragm of the stethoscope, listen for bowel sounds: the frequency, pitch, quality and pattern. Frequent, tinkling high-pitched runs are heard in bowel obstruction. Bowel sounds will be absent in ileus or peritonitis. Auscultation over the liver edge as a finger gently scratches from the abdomen to the chest is useful to define the liver edge; you can also listen for

the (rare) hepatic bruit of a hepatoma.

Vascular bruits of the femoral arteries in the groin or renal arteries may be heard. A renal bruit is best

heard by listening posteriorly over the renal angle between the spine and the 12th rib (position ① and ② in Fig. 5.6) with the patient sitting up.

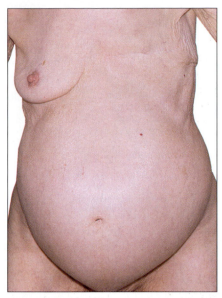

Fig. 5.5 Malignant ascites from metastatic breast cancer

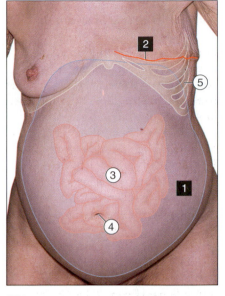

KEY
▮1 Distended abdomen (fluid, dull to percussion)
▮2 Mastectomy scar
③ Bowel (resonant to percussion)
④ Umbilicus
⑤ Ribs

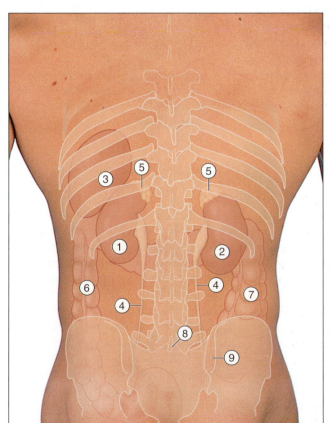

KEY
① Left kidney
② Right kidney
③ Spleen
④ Ureter
⑤ Adrenal glands
⑥ Descending colon
⑦ Ascending colon
⑧ 5th lumbar spine
⑨ Posterior superior iliac spine

Fig. 5.6 Posterior abdominal wall: bones and soft tissue

Investigations

The list of possible investigations for abdominal symptoms is extensive. Depending on the symptoms and signs a key test may confirm the diagnosis (Table 5.1). The following investigations may also be useful:

- Urine testing for pH, specific gravity, blood, protein, urobilinogen
- Pregnancy testing of urine (for βHCG)
- Faecal occult blood testing
- Haematology: haemoglobin, mean corpuscular volume (MCV), white cell count with differential count, blood film, vitamin B$_{12}$, folate, international normalized ratio (INR), partial thromboplastin time kaolin (PTTK), supplementary tests of the clotting cascade
- Erythrocyte sedimentation rate (ESR), plasma viscosity and C-reactive protein
- Biochemistry: urea, sodium, potassium, chloride, creatinine, liver function tests, amylase, serum tumour markers (CEA, CA125, CA153)
- Arterial blood gases P_{O_2}, P_{CO_2}, bicarbonate, hydrogen ion, base excess
- Radiology: plain erect chest and supine abdominal radiographs, ultrasound, single or double contrast radiology, intravenous urogram, isotope renal scan, CT scanning (with contrast), MRI scanning, interventional techniques including percutaneous transhepatic cholangiography, angiography
- Endoscopy (with biopsy where appropriate): upper gastrointestinal endoscopy, endoscopic ultrasound, enteroscopy, endoscopic retrograde cholangiopancreatography (ERCP), proctoscopy, rigid or flexible sigmoidoscopy, colonoscopy
- Laparoscopy (with peritoneal lavage or biopsy), laparoscopic ultrasound
- Biopsy by fine needle, core or open incisional/excisional techniques.

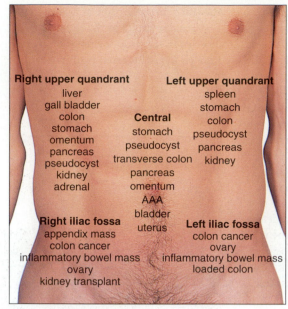

Fig. 5.7 Anatomical structures in relation to the overlying abdominal wall

Right upper quandrant
liver
gall bladder
colon
stomach
omentum
pancreas
pseudocyst
kidney
adrenal

Left upper quandrant
spleen
stomach
colon
pseudocyst
pancreas
kidney

Central
stomach
pseudocyst
transverse colon
pancreas
omentum
AAA
bladder
uterus

Right iliac fossa
appendix mass
colon cancer
inflammatory bowel mass
ovary
kidney transplant

Left iliac fossa
colon cancer
ovary
inflammatory bowel mass
loaded colon

Table 5.1 Common causes of abdominal pain

Condition	Typical features	Key investigation
Biliary colic	Upper abdominal pain, increasing to plateau and dispersing after a few hours; may be described as a band around the upper (right) abdomen	Ultrasound
Pancreatitis	*Acute:* severe epigastric pain, radiating to back; may imitate peptic ulcer	Serum/urine amylase
	Chronic: persistent abdominal/back pain, with exacerbations; features of pancreatic insufficiency	ERCP
Peptic ulcer	Dyspepsia; epigastric pain, worse or relieved on eating; patient wakens at night	Upper endoscopy
Renal colic	Severe right/left-sided pain radiating to the groin/testicle	Intravenous urogram
Colonic neoplasm	Rectal bleeding; anaemia; mucus; change in bowel habit	Colonoscopy
Diverticular disease	Left iliac fossa pain; pellet stools; diarrhoea/constipation; rectal bleeding	Barium enema
Bowel obstruction	Abdominal distension; colicky pain; vomiting	Plain radiograph

ACUTE UPPER ABDOMEN

The cause of an acute abdomen differs according to the age and gender of the individual. Remember that significant conditions above the diaphragm – myocardial ischaemia or infarction, pneumonia, lung infarction – can present with upper abdominal pain.

Pancreatitis

History

Pancreatitis may be acute or chronic and is usually secondary to alcohol or gallstones (Table 5.2). Thus ask about a history of alcohol ingestion and whether there are known gallstones. The pain of pancreatitis is classically epigastric and radiates to the back, so, in contrast to a perforated peptic ulcer, it may be eased by sitting forwards or by moving around. Other causes of pancreatitis which may be evident from the history (Table 5.2) are medications, hypercholesterolaemia or ERCP (iatrogenic pancreatitis). Ask about the duration and severity of the pain, whether there have been previous episodes, and about associated features which may signal respiratory or renal compromise such as breath-

Table 5.2 Causes of pancreatitis

Frequency	Cause
Common (80% of cases in UK)	Gallstones Alcohol
Intermediate	Trauma (post-ERCP, blunt abdominal trauma) Tumour (ampullary or pancreatic) Drugs (e.g, azathioprine, beta-blockers, steroids) Infection (e.g. viruses, particularly mumps) Hyperlipidaemias Hypothermia
Rare	Metabolic (e.g. hypercalcaemia) Congenital (e.g. pancreas divisum)
10% of cases	Idiopathic

Table 5.3 Early prognostic criteria for severity of acute pancreatitis

Criterion	Threshold
Age of patient	>55 years
White blood cells	>15 ×10⁹/l
Glucose (in blood)	>10 mmol/l
Urea	>16 mmol/l
Pao_2	<8 kPa
Calcium	<2.0 mmol/l
Albumin	<32 g/l
LDH (lactate dehydrogenase)	>600 iu/l
ALT (alanine aminotransferase)	>100 iu/l

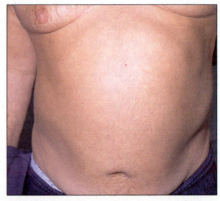

Fig. 5.8 Acute panctreatitis

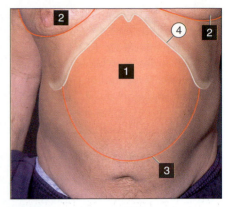

KEY

1 Tender area
2 Gynaecomastia
3 Epigastric mass
④ Rib margin

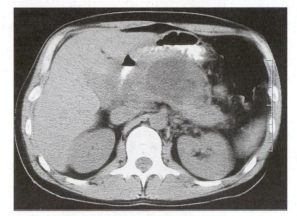

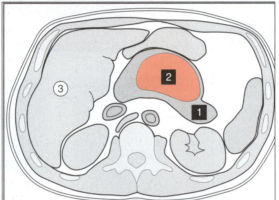

KEY

1 Inflamed pancreas
2 Pancreatic pseudocyst
③ Liver

Fig. 5.9 CT scan in acute pancreatitis

lessness, poor urinary output, thirst, nausea or vomiting. For chronic pancreatitis, ask about the number and severity of previous episodes, use of analgesics between episodes and indicators of failing exocrine pancreatic function (steatorrhoea, weight loss) or endocrine function (diabetes).

Examination

On **inspection**, look for signs of malnutrition or liver disease (associated with alcoholic pancreatitis) such as gynaecomastia (Fig. 5.8 2). Periumbilical or flank bruising are rare signs of acute pancreatitis, but peripheral oedema (hypoalbuminaemia) is more common. The patient may be breathless because of the abdominal contents splinting the diaphragm or pleural effusions. Erythema ab igne may indicate chronic use of a hot water bottle to lessen the pain (Fig. 5.10).

Palpation may be tender in the epigastrium (Fig. 5.8 1) and may reveal a central abdominal inflammatory mass 3 or, following acute pancreatitis, a pseudocyst (Fig. 5.9 2) (a collection of fluid trapped in the retroperitoneum).

Percussion to detect shifting dullness may elicit ascites (Fig. 5.5).

Auscultation may fail to hear bowel sounds in acute pancreatitis. Chest examination for pulmonary signs and pleural effusion (p. 21) is commonly positive in acute pancreatitis.

Investigations

A serum amylase three times the upper limit of normal is diagnostic of acute pancreatitis. Other blood tests are used to indicate the severity of the attack. These criteria comprise haematological and biochemical indices which together with the patient's age can be used to predict the severity of the attack (Table 5.3).

To investigate the cause of acute

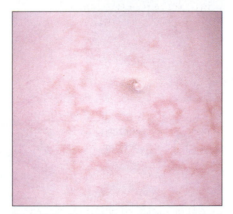

Fig. 5.10 Erythema ab igne – chronic abdominal pain relieved by a hot water bottle, damaging the skin

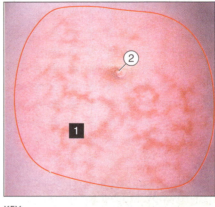

KEY

1 Erythema ab igne   ② Umbilicus

pancreatitis, ultrasound may usefully demonstrate gallstones (Fig. 5.14) which if multiple and small may have migrated down the biliary tree to

cause the pancreatitis. CT scanning may demonstrate an inflamed pancreas (Fig. 5.9), peripancreatic oedema, pancreatic necrosis and/or a pseudocyst **2**, and any pulmonary collapse or effusions. In acute gallstone pancreatitis, ERCP and sphincterotomy may be diagnostic and therapeutic. If alcohol or gallstones are not responsible, raised lipids and viral titres may suggest the cause.

Management

Management is usually supportive, with oxygen, fluids and analgesia to prevent and treat respiratory, renal and cardiac complications. Intra-abdominal complications may require surgical intervention.

Perforated peptic ulcer

Perforated duodenal (Fig. 5.11 **3**) or gastric ulcer presents as a sudden onset of severe epigastric pain quickly spreading across the whole abdomen as peritoneal soiling with lumenal contents occurs **4**. The patient holds the abdomen rigid to stop movement further irritating the inflamed peritoneum. There may be a preceding history of epigastric burning or pain typically relieved by food. Particularly in the elderly population, NSAIDs may be responsible for the peptic ulcer.

In contrast to pancreatitis, remaining very still is most comfortable and movement exacerbates the pain.

Examination

On **inspection**, the patient will usually be lying still, on his back, taking shallow breaths, and may have a pale, sweaty face. Gentle **palpation** of the abdomen will demonstrate a board-like rigidity (guarding), and even gentle **percussion** (for rebound) may be painful. **Auscultation** for bowel sounds will be silent once chemical, then bacterial, peritonitis is established.

Investigations and treatment

A raised white cell count and slightly elevated amylase may support the diagnosis. An erect PA chest radiograph (Fig. 5.12) shows free air **1** under the diaphragm **2** in 70% of patients with a perforated peptic ulcer (Fig. 5.11 **3**). If no free air is seen and the diagnosis is in doubt, a water soluble contrast meal may show flow of contrast into the peritoneal cavity. Laparoscopy, at least for some perforated peptic ulcers, may visually demonstrate the perforation and allow closure and lavage by laparoscopic or open techniques.

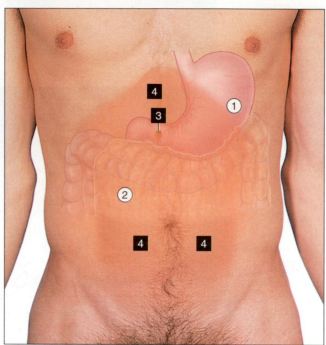

KEY
(1) Stomach
(2) Greater omentum
3 Anterior duodenal perforation
4 Extent of pertoneal soiling

Fig. 5.11 Perforated anterior duodenal ulcer showing extent of initial peritoneal soiling

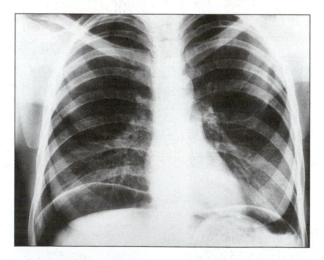

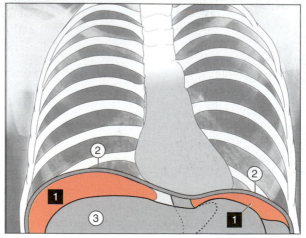

KEY
1 Free intraperitoneal air
(2) Diaphragm
(3) Liver

Fig. 5.12 Erect chest radiograph in a patient with a perforated peptic ulcer

Acute cholecystitis

Acute cholecystitis presents as progressive, increasing, constant right upper quadrant (Fig. 5.13 **2**) or epigastric pain, which may radiate to the back or be associated with shoulder tip pain. Nausea and vomiting may also occur. There may be a history of indigestion or previous similar painful episodes lasting a few hours.

Examination

On **inspection**, the patient will lie still, may be pyrexial and, in the less common situation where a gallstone has also migrated down the biliary tree, may be jaundiced (Fig. 5.3). There may be a visible mass (Fig. 5.13 **1**) in the right upper quadrant, particularly if the acute cholecystitis has led to an inflammatory mass of omentum gathering around the gall bladder, or an empyema. Gentle **palpation** will demonstrate tenderness in the right upper quadrant **2** and epigastrium, and may reveal a palpable mass.

Murphy's sign, which refers to the way in which a patient catches his breath on inspiration when firm pressure is applied over the gall bladder at the costal margin, is a good indicator of acute cholecystitis. Courvoisier's law states that if the gall bladder is palpable in a jaundiced patient then the jaundice is not likely to be due to gallstones (i.e. gallstones are usually found in small, thick-walled and shrunken gall bladders).

Percussion over the right upper quadrant will elicit rebound tenderness. **Auscultation** should reveal normal bowel sounds.

Investigation

A raised white cell count is common and mild derangement of liver function tests (LFTs) or amylase may occur in acute cholecystitis. The key investigation is ultrasound (Fig. 5.14), which may demonstrate a thick-walled gall bladder containing gallstones **1**, often with surrounding oedema. The biliary tree may also be examined to see whether there is any associated duct dilatation from migrating stones (which may result in grossly abnormal LFTs).

Treatment

Treatment of the acute episode may include antibiotics with subsequent laparoscopic cholecystectomy to remove the stone-bearing gall bladder **3**, or removal of the acutely inflamed gall bladder at the same admission.

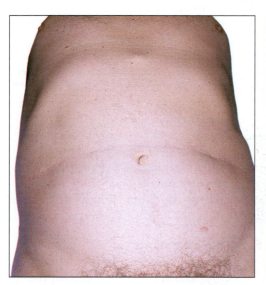
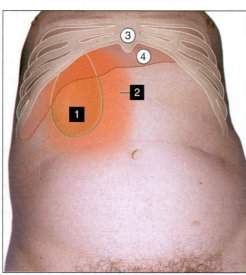
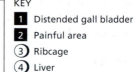

KEY
1 Distended gall bladder
2 Painful area
3 Ribcage
4 Liver

Fig. 5.13 Acute cholecystitis, which has developed into empyema of the gall bladder

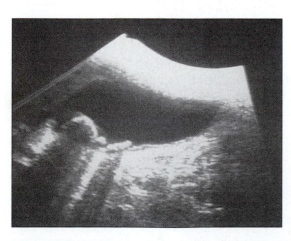
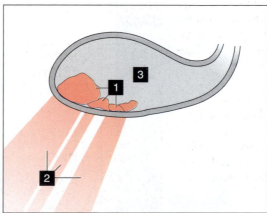

KEY
1 Gallstones
2 Acoustic shadow
3 Gall bladder

Fig. 5.14 Ultrasound appearance in gallstone disease

Hepatomegaly and jaundice

History

Ask about jaundice (Fig. 5.3), itch, bruising, dark urine, pale stools, pain, fever, bowel habit, and prodromal symptoms. A past history of foreign travel, blood transfusion, tattoos, drug usage (recreational or pre-scribed), alcohol intake, occupation, previous surgical and medical illnesses (including surgical resections for cancer), a sexual history and a family history are all important. Common causes of hepatomegaly include cardiac failure, metastatic cancer and infection.

Examination

Inspect to see if the patient is jaundiced or has stigmata of liver disease, which may include palmar erythema, Dupuytren's contractures, finger clubbing (Fig. 3.2), spider naevi, gynaecomastia (Fig. 5.8), bruising, peripheral oedema, testicular atrophy, sparse body hair, and flapping tremor. Look also for signs of right heart failure, including a raised jugulo-venous pressure (JVP) and peripheral oedema. Inspect the abdomen to look for surgical scars, scratch marks, stretch marks or a distended abdomen (ascites, Fig. 5.5), dilated veins or a mass in the right upper quadrant.

To **palpate** the edge of the liver (Fig. 5.15 ③), start in the right iliac fossa and palpate towards the right costal margin, using the tips of your fingers gently applied to the abdominal wall as you ask the patient to breathe in deeply. The edge of the

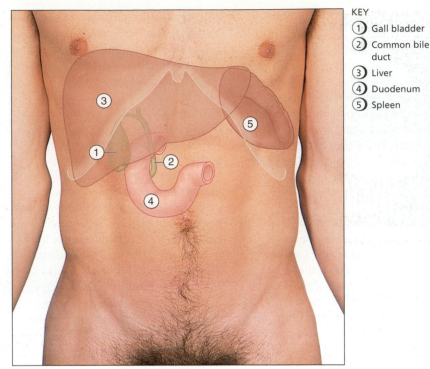

Fig. 5.15 Hepatobiliary tract and associated structures

KEY
① Gall bladder
② Common bile duct
③ Liver
④ Duodenum
⑤ Spleen

liver, if palpable, will move inferiorly with each deep inspiration and will meet your fingers. Using this palpation technique, you can define the lower border of the liver and state how many centimetres below the costal margin it lies and the nature of the liver edge (smooth/craggy, tender/non-tender), pulsatile (suggesting tricuspid regurgitation) or hard (tumour, Fig. 5.16)). To palpate for enlarged spleen (Fig. 5.15 ⑤), which may be associated with hepatomegaly, again start in the *right* iliac fossa, palpating using the pulps of your fingers, moving in towards the left costal margin with deep inspiration.

Using **percussion**, percuss the lower, then upper, border of the liver (which should lie in the fourth intercostal space in the midclavicular line, Fig. 5.15 ③). Percuss for shifting dullness.

Using **auscultation**, place the stethoscope over the lower border of the liver and draw your index finger across the skin, passing from the gas containing abdomen onto the solid liver, listening for a change in the quality and the pitch of the sound. Listen also for the bruit of a hepatoma (Fig. 5.17).

Investigations

Urine should be tested for bilirubin (present in the urine in posthepatic and hepatic jaundice) and urobilinogen

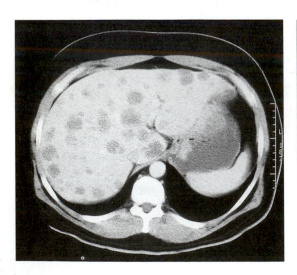

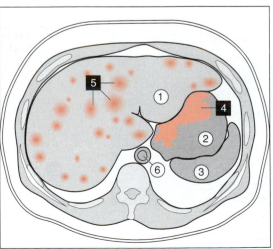

KEY
① Liver
② Stomach
③ Spleen
④ Gastric cancer
⑤ Multiple liver metastases
⑥ Aorta

Fig. 5.16 CT scan through the liver and stomach demonstrating primary and metastatic gastric cancer

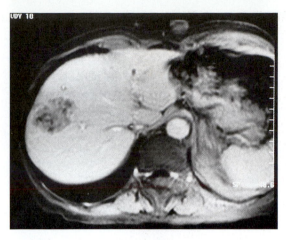

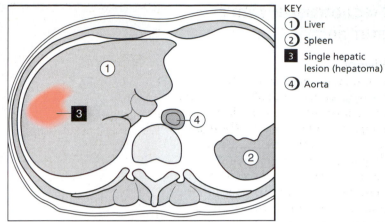

Fig. 5.17 MRI scan showing a hepatoma

(present in the urine in prehepatic jaundice) (Fig. 5.18).

Blood tests may detect abnormal coagulation (prothrombin time), anaemia, raised white cell count, raised platelet count, low sodium, deranged urea and potassium, low albumin and elevated LFTs: alanine aminotransferase (ALT), alkaline phosphatase, gamma glutamyl transferase (GGT), bilirubin, alpha fetoprotein (raised in hepatoma) or carcinoembryonic antigen (CEA) (raised in colorectal liver metastases). The differential elevation of liver function tests in a jaundiced patient (Table 5.4) can be helpful in suggesting a diagnosis.

Ultrasound scanning for gallstones (Fig. 5.14), liver size and texture, hepatic lesions, and dilated bile ducts may be supplemented by a contrast enhanced CT scan (Fig. 5.16) or MRI scan (Fig. 5.17).

Needle aspiration of a sample of ascitic fluid or biopsy of the liver under radiological or laparoscopic guidance can establish the histological diagnosis.

Treatment

Treatment of jaundice or hepatomegaly is aimed at the underlying cause.

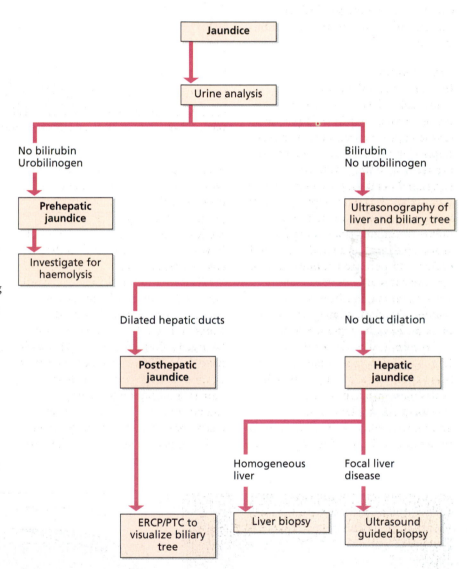

Fig. 5.18 Investigations for jaundice

Table 5.4 Liver function tests in a jaundiced patient		
Jaundice type	**Test**	**Result**
Hepatic jaundice	Bilirubin	↑↑↑
	ALT	↑↑↑
	GGT	↑↑↑
	Alk phos	↑
Obstructive jaundice	Bilirubin	↑↑↑
	ALT	↑
	GGT	↑
	Alk phos	↑↑↑

Oesophageal cancer and gastric cancer

History

Oesophageal and gastric cancer (Fig. 5.19 **2** and Fig. 5.21 **2**) develop in the mucosa of the oesophagus or stomach respectively, impinge on the lumen (Fig. 5.20 ②)and spread to involve local structures and lymph nodes outwith the wall of the oesophagus and stomach. The history should include a full gastrointestinal enquiry. Is there dysphagia – for solids (usually meat first), semisolids, liquids or even total dysphagia? If vomiting occurs, how soon is it after ingestion – immediate (i.e. regurgitation), partly digested food, previous meals (implying gastric outlet obstruction)? What colour is the vomit? Is there any blood in the vomitus? Weight loss (how much over what time period, or changes in size of clothing) and anorexia are key features of more advanced disease. Conversely, anaemia causing breathlessness or melaena from more acute blood loss may occur even in early disease.

Are there symptoms of spread, e.g. hoarseness (due to recurrent laryngeal nerve palsy), breathlessness (aspiration pneumonia or pneumonia secondary to occlusion of a bronchus by metastatic disease, malignant pleural effusion) or metastasis to the liver (Fig. 5.16) or bones?

A general medical history is important in assessing fitness for operative treatment – many patients have cardiorespiratory diseases. Squamous oesophageal cancer affects the middle third of the oesophagus and is strongly linked to tobacco and alcohol usage. Lower oesophageal cancer (especially that occurring in Barrett's metaplastic oesophagus) is usually an adenocarcinoma (Fig. 5.20 **1**). In the stomach, 95% of cancers are adenocarcinoma.

Examination

Does the patient appear to be well nourished or cachectic, pale or jaundiced? Examine the hands for signs of loss of muscle mass, pallor, or leuconychia.

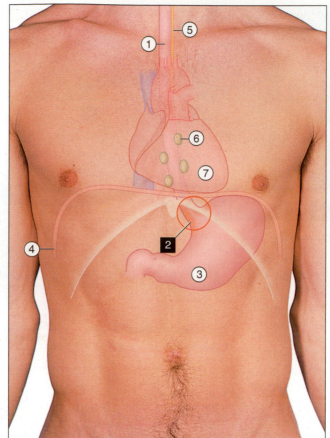

KEY
① Oesophagus
2 Site of lower oesophageal cancer
③ Stomach
④ Diaphragm
⑤ Recurrent laryngeal nerve
⑥ Mediastinal nodes to which oesophageal cancer may drain
⑦ Heart

Fig. 5.19 Position of oesophogastric junction cancer and relation to intrathoracic structures (see Fig. 5.22 for relevant intra-abdominal structures)

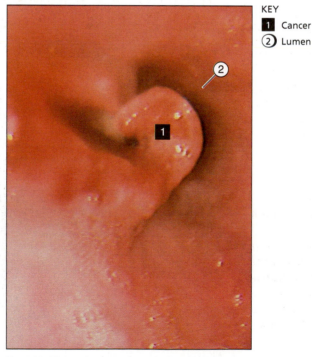

KEY
1 Cancer
② Lumen

Fig. 5.20 Obstructing oesophageal adenocarcinoma

Inspection of the abdomen typically confirms recent weight loss and may suggest an epigastric mass or ascites. Check for a succussion splash where gastric outflow obstruction (due to an antral cancer, see Fig. 5.21 2) results in a large resting collection of fluid in the stomach. **Palpate** for a non tender upper abdominal mass which may be associated with hepatomegaly (due to metastatic disease). **Percuss** for the shifting dullness of ascites (Fig. 5.5). **Auscultation** does not usually help in the diagnosis.

Investigations

- Haemoglobin for anaemia, raised ESR/plasma viscosity
- White cell count for infective complications
- Electrolytes (particularly looking for low potassium, low chloride in chronic vomiting).

Radiology. Chest radiography may demonstrates metastases, pleural effusion or signs of aspiration pneumonia. Ultrasound or CT scanning (chest/abdomen) is used to assess the extent of the cancer and the presence of node or liver metastases or ascites. Fibreoptic endoscopy is the key investigation (Fig. 5.22) with biopsy, this will not only allow the precise location and size of the cancer 2 to be measured but also biopsy for histological diagnosis. A barium swallow (Fig. 5.23) may be useful to delineate the length of an oesophageal cancer. Endoscopic ultrasound can show the depth of tumour invasion. Laparoscopy can be used to decide if a cancer is likely to be resectable.

Management

Most oesophageal and gastric cancers present at a late stage; surgical removal can be curative in a minority. Alternatively, perioperative chemotherapy or chemoradiotherapy may improve the prognosis. Stenting (placing a tube through the cancer) allows a patient to swallow. Laser therapy, radiotherapy, or chemo-therapy may be used to palliate the cancer.

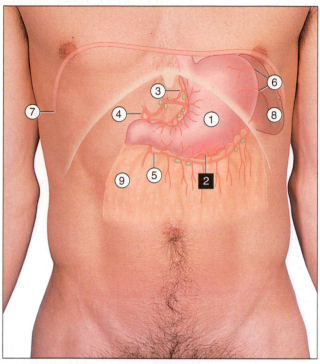

KEY
1. Stomach
2. Site of gastric cancer
3. Left gastric artery
4. Right gastric artery
5. Gastroepiploic artery
6. Short gastric vessels
7. Diaphragm
8. Spleen
9. Greater omentum

Fig. 5.21 Gastric cancer showing arterial blood supply and lymph node drainage

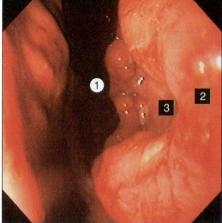

KEY
1. Endoscope
2. Cancer
3. Ulcerated cancer

Fig. 5.22 Endoscopic view of ulcerated gastric cancer

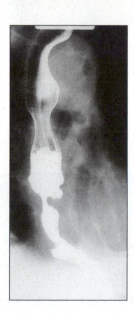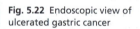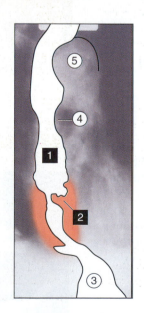

KEY
1. Dilated oesophagus
2. Cancer
3. Stomach
4. Peristaltic wave
5. Arch of aorta

Fig. 5.23 Barium swallow showing oesophageal cancer

ACUTE LOWER ABDOMEN

Aneurysm

History

Abdominal aortic aneurysm (AAA) (Fig. 5.25 **1**, Fig. 5.26 **1**) may be entirely asymptomatic or cause backache. However, a leaking aneurysm (usually the leak is retroperitoneal) causes severe back pain which may be one sided and radiate to the groin, and thus cause confusion with renal colic. However, aneurysm disease develops after the age of 50, whereas renal colic usually occurs under 40 years old. The aneurysm may occlude the inferior mesenteric artery (Fig. 5.24 ⑨) causing colonic ischaemia, or the renal arteries ⑦ causing hypertension or loss of renal function. A leaking aneurysm may be associated with symptoms (fainting, sweating, feeling cold) and signs (postural hypotension, tachycardia) of acute blood loss. There may be a history of peripheral or cardiac vascular disease, often associated with smoking. Ask about past medical history, medications, and associated cardiorespiratory diseases.

Examination

A leaking aneurysm may present with the classic features of shock (due to blood loss) – pallor, sweating, altered conscious level – and is a real surgical emergency. Outwith this emergency situation, look for outward signs of cardiorespiratory disease and smoking. On **inspection** of the abdomen, a pulsation may be visible. **Palpate** for an expansile mass adjacent to the umbilicus (Fig. 5.25 **1** and ④): place your index fingers parallel, gently pressing either side of the aorta and feel them being pushed apart. It may be possible to assess the size of the aneurysm in centimetres. The normal aorta may be palpable in a thin individual where the pulsation is transmitted to the abdominal wall. Palpation of the femoral arteries may reveal an absent pulse. **Percussion** is not useful but on **auscultation** you may hear a bruit secondary to disturbed blood flow in the aorta or the femoral or renal arteries.

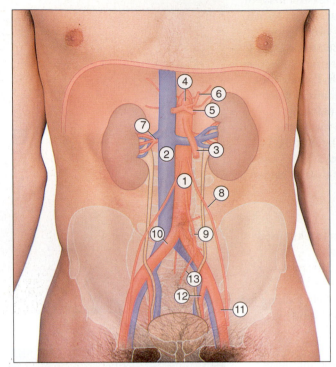

Fig. 5.24 Arterial anatomy of the abdomen

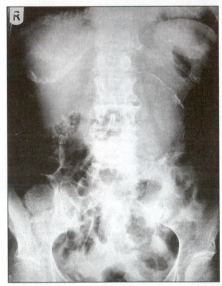

Fig. 5.25 Plain radiograph of abdominal aortic dissection

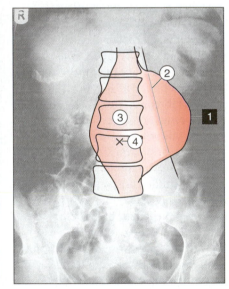

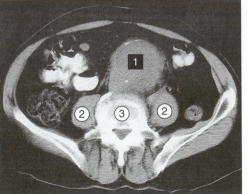

Fig. 5.26 CT scan of abdominal aortic aneurysm

Investigation

The key investigation is a CT scan (Fig. 5.26) to map the size and extent of the aneurysm **1** and the presence of a leak. Ultrasound scanning is useful to document the size of an aneurysm found electively.

A full blood count for anaemia and raised white cell count is indicated in the acute situation. Measurement of urea and creatinine levels may reveal reduced renal function in both acute and chronic presentations of an aneurysm (the aneurysm may involve the origin of the renal arteries).

Management

Elective replacement of the aneurysmal segment by placing a graft in the aorta at open surgery or using a radiologically placed stent is usually advised for aneurysms of 5 cm or greater. Emergency replacement of a leaking aneurysm is a true surgical emergency with a high mortality.

Renal colic

A classic history of renal colic is the rapid onset of unilateral loin pain radiating into the groin (and in males to the testis) on the same side. The pain is usually due to a small stone passing from the renal pelvis (Fig. 5.27 ③) down the ureter ④, driven on by waves of ureteric peristalsis (hence the waves of colicky pain). The pain is usually sufficiently severe to elicit nausea and vomiting, pallor and sweating, but unlike many causes of acute abdominal pain, may be more bearable if the patient moves around. There may be a history of previous similar episodes, relieved by analgesia (NSAIDs are as effective as opiates). Ask about a history of living or working in hot conditions, excess milk ingestion or a family history of stone disease. Urinary tract stones may be associated with urinary tract infections or known anatomical variants.

Examination

On **inspection**, the patient may be pale, sweating, restless and, if there is also urinary tract infection, pyrexial. **Palpation** of the abdomen may identify renal angle tenderness, tenderness in the iliac fossa of the affected side but no rebound or guarding. **Percussion** and **auscultation** are not usually helpful.

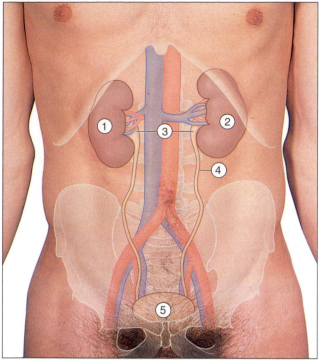

KEY
① Right kidney
② Left kidney
③ Renal pelvis
④ Ureter
⑤ Bladder

Fig. 5.27 Normal anatomy of urinary system

Investigations

Urinary testing and microscopy will demonstrate microscopic haematuria and protein, and may show crystals. Blood testing shows a raised white cell count, though usually biochemistry is normal. Plain abdominal radiology may let you identify a stone in the line of the ureter ④ or additional stones in the renal pelvis ③ or bladder ⑤. Intravenous urography (Fig. 5.28) of intravenous contrast excreted by the kidneys very effectively outlines the upper urinary tract **1** **2** and may delineate a stone obstructing the ureter **3**.

Management

Most stones pass from the ureter unaided into the bladder and so analgesia is the main treatment. Some stones lodge, usually as the ureter passes through the bladder wall **3**, and require lithotriptic destruction or endoscopic removal.

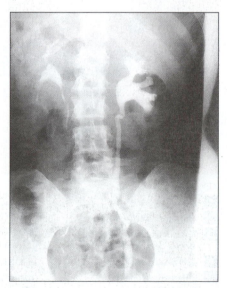

Fig. 5.28 Intravenous urogram

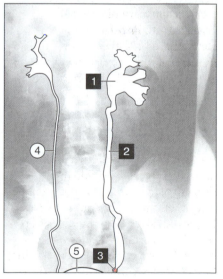

KEY
1 Dilated renal pelvis
2 Dilated ureter
3 Stone
④ Normal urinary tract
⑤ Bladder

Appendicitis

Appendicitis typically occurs between the ages of 10 and 30, but children and the elderly can also have appendicitis and may cause particular diagnostic difficulties.

History

The typical history of appendicitis is of progressive onset of colicky central abdominal pain (Fig. 5.29a). This moves to become a localized pain in the right iliac fossa (Fig. 5.29b) over McBurney's point ③ (a point ²/₃ along a line between the umbilicus ① and the anterior superior iliac spine ②) as the peritoneum of the abdom-inal wall becomes involved in the inflammatory process. Associated features may include anorexia; initially, there may be vomiting and a loose bowel motion. Because of the extensive differential diagnosis (Fig. 5.30 and Table 5.5), ask about a recent upper respiratory tract infection (which may be associated with mesenteric adenitis (Fig. 5.30 ■1■)), urinary symptoms ■8■ (which may also occur in appendicitis with irritation of the bladder by the appendix) and in females aged 10–60 take a careful menstrual history.

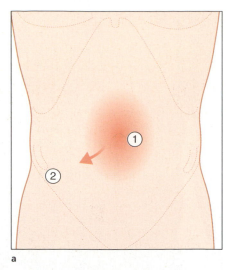
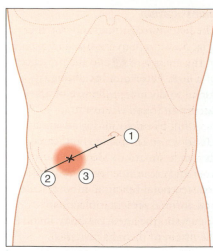

Fig. 5.29 In appendicitis progressive onset of colicky central abdominal pain (**a**) moving to become a localized pain in the right iliac fossa (**b**) deep to McBurney's point

KEY
① Umbilicus
② Anterior superior iliac spine
③ X = McBurney's point

Table 5.4 Differential diagnosis of appendicitis
Mesenteric adenitis (Fig. 5.30 ■1■)
Gynaecological conditions (including ectopic pregnancy ■7■ , pelvic inflammatory disease ■5■)
Ovarian pathology ■6■
Urinary tract infection ■8■
Infective gastrointestinal tract conditions
Inflammatory bowel disease ■3■
Meckel's diverticulitis ■2■
Caecal cancer ■4■

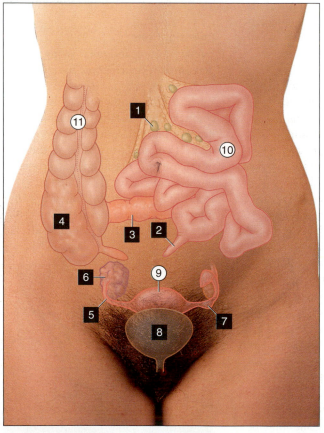

Fig. 5.30 Differential diagnosis of appendicitis

KEY
■1■ Mesenteric adenitis
■2■ Meckel's diverticulitis
■3■ Terminal ileum inflammatory bowel disease
■4■ Caecal cancer
■5■ Inflamed fallopian tube/fimbria
■6■ Ovarian cyst – or torted ovary
■7■ Ectopic pregnancy
■8■ Bladder infection
⑨ Uterus
⑩ Ileum
⑪ Ascending colon

Examination

On examination, the patient will be lying still and may have a slight pyrexia (typically 37.5°C).

On **inspection** of the abdomen, a long-standing appendicitis which has been walled off by omentum or developed into a right iliac fossa abscess may be visible in a thin person as a right iliac fossa mass. Look for scars of previous surgery. On gentle then deeper **palpation**, an established appendicitis will be evident as localized tenderness with rebound and guarding in the right iliac fossa (Fig. 5.29b). An appendix mass may be delineated by gentle palpation. **Percussion** will elicit rebound and **auscultation** normal bowel sounds unless the appendicitis has developed into a generalized peritonitis.

Investigations and treatment

All blood tests may be normal although, as the inflammatory process proceeds, a raised white cell count and raised C-reactive protein (CRP) should occur. Ultrasound of the right iliac fossa may demonstrate an omental mass or abscess if presenting late or identify gynaecological conditions (Fig. 5.30). Test the urine to exclude a urinary tract infection (blood, protein) or pregnancy (test for βHCG in the urine). In theatre, under general anaesthesia, laparoscopy in women of child-bearing age can be extremely useful if the diagnosis is in doubt. The treatment of acute appendicitis is surgical excision through an incision in the right iliac fossa usually centred on McBurney's point (Fig. 5.29b ③) two-thirds of the way along a line from the umbilicus to the anterior superior iliac spine.

Intra-abdominal sepsis from acute appendicitis (or perforated peptic ulcer, inflammatory bowel disease or diverticular disease) may localize in any one of several loci within the peritoneum (Fig. 5.31). Treatment of such abscesses usually requires surgical drainage and peritoneal lavage.

Meckel's diverticulum (a remnant of the embryo vitello-intestinal tract) may become inflamed (Fig. 5.32 **1**) initiating acute appendicitis. It may be excised.

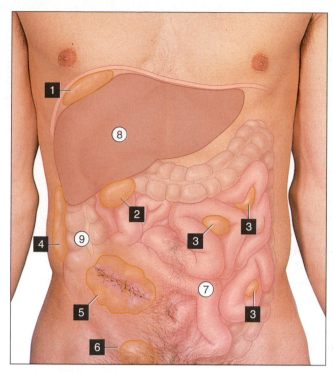

Fig. 5.31 Abdominal complications of appendicitis

KEY
1 Subphrenic abscess
2 Subhepatic abscess
3 Interloop abscesses
4 Paracolic gutter abscess
5 Wound abscess
6 Pelvic abscess
⑦ Small bowel
⑧ Liver
⑨ Colon

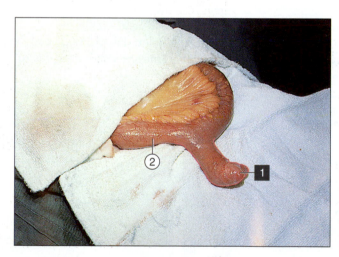

Fig. 5.32 Meckel's diverticulitis in a patient originally thought to have appendicitis

KEY
1 Meckel's diverticulum with Meckel's diverticulitis at tip
② Terminal ileum

Inflammatory bowel disease

History

Inflammatory bowel disease (Crohn's disease, ulcerative colitis) has a chronic course with relapses and remissions and often requires surgical assessment. A detailed history will include the number of episodes, age when they started, usual course of acute events, medications, dietary modifications/supplementation and/or operations required.

Questions about gastrointestinal symptoms should obtain information about mouth ulcers, dysphagia, abdominal pain (upper, central or lower abdominal pain which may or may not be well localized), nausea, vomiting, diarrhoea (with blood or mucus), constipation, abdominal masses, jaundice/itch (related to hepatobiliary disease), fistulae to the abdominal wall, perianal abscesses, and anal fistulae. Other (systemic) manifestations relate to eye symptoms, skin rashes (erythema nodosum or pyoderma gangrenosum), arthropathies, and weight loss.

There may be a family history of inflammatory bowel disease.

Examination

On **inspection**, look for signs of malnutrition, pallor, jaundice or itch and, in an acute episode, pyrexia. On inspection of the abdomen, look for previous scars, stoma, fistulae, and obvious masses. Anal and digital rectal examination should note scars, abscesses, fistulae or blood on the gloved finger.

Superficial then deep **palpation** may reveal one or more abdominal masses and may be tender. A palpable mass can also be delineated by **percussion**. In acute colitis, the transverse colon (Fig. 5.33 ⑥) and caecum ④ may be very tender, due to dilation, even on light percussion. On **auscultation**, the bowel sounds may be normal or there may be signs of small or large bowel obstruction (see pp. 52–54).

The signs, like the symptoms, for inflammatory bowel disease are highly variable; involvement of parietal peritoneum in the inflammatory process (Figs 5.34, 5.35) should be compared with the normal surface anatomy (Fig. 5.33).

KEY
1. Ileum
2. Terminal ileum
3. Appendix
4. Caecum
5. Ascending colon
6. Transverse colon
7. Descending colon
8. Sigmoid colon
9. Upper rectum

Fig. 5.33 Normal colon anatomy

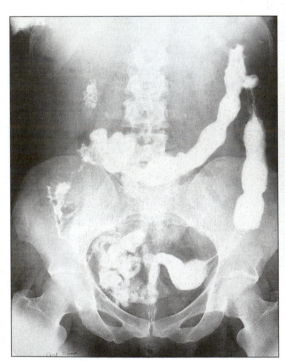
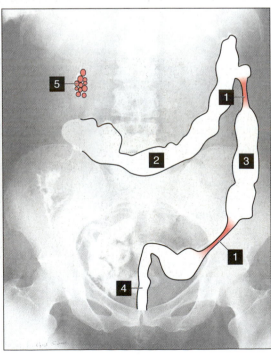

KEY
1. Colonic strictures
2. Transverse colon
3. Descending colon
4. Rectum
5. Radiopaque gallstones (incidental finding)

Fig. 5.34 Contrast enema showing Crohn's disease of the colon with stricture formation ▮1

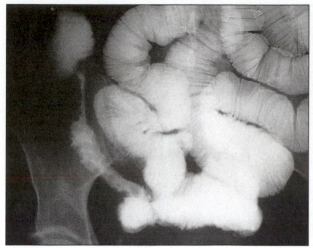

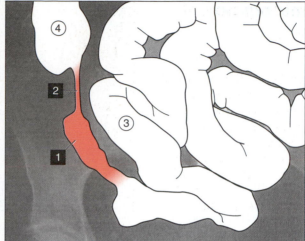

Fig. 5.35 Contrast follow through showing inflammation and stricture of the terminal ileum in Crohn's disease.

KEY

1 Inflamed terminal ileum showing mucosal oedema
2 Stricture of terminal ileum (Crohn's disease)
③ Normal small bowel
④ Caecum

Investigation

A raised white cell count and CRP are associated with acute and ongoing chronic inflammatory processes. There may be anaemia due to ongoing blood loss or malabsorption of vitamin B_{12}, folate or iron. Blood biochemistry can detect evidence of hepatic disturbance (deranged LFTs), and low albumin due to malnutrition and/or liver disease. Plain abdominal films may show dilated small bowel secondary to obstruction by stricture (e.g. Fig. 5.35) or dilated colon due to acute ulcerative colitis. Progressive dilatation of the colon may result in toxic megacolon, where the colon

becomes dilated, ischaemic and per- forates resulting in shock then death. Contrast radiology can be extremely useful in delineating the extent of small intestinal (Fig. 5.35) and colonic (Fig. 5.34) disease, internal and ex- ternal fistulae (Fig. 5.36) and sclerosing cholangitis. Ultrasound, CT or MRI can be used to detect intra-abdominal collections. MRI can provide detailed maps of perianal fistulae.

Gentle per anal examination, proctoscopy, sigmoidoscopy and colonoscopy allow direct inspection of the rectal and colonic mucosa for ulcerative colitis or Crohn's disease with biopsy where appropriate. If

(rare) upper gastro-intestinal tract Crohn's disease is suspected upper endoscopy may be helpful.

Management

Management includes medical manage- ment of inflammatory bowel and systemic manifestations with immuno- suppressants and steroids in a tablet or enema form, together with dietary and nutritional support. Surgical intervention for individual problems – abscess, strictures, obstruction, fistula (Fig. 5.36), supervening carcinoma of the colon – is conducted on an individualized basis.

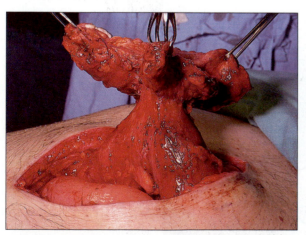

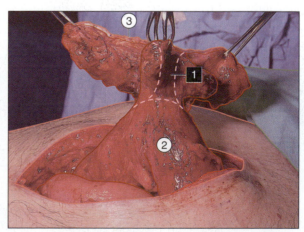

KEY

1 Fistula
② Ileum
③ Skin

Fig. 5.36 Excision of fistula to site of previous surgery caused by Crohn's disease.

Ischaemic bowel

History

Ischaemic small intestine occurs as chronic ischaemia (central abdominal pain after food) or as sudden onset of severe pain from acute mesenteric ischaemia then infarction, usually affecting the whole small bowel due to occlusion of the superior mesenteric artery (Fig. 5.37). Colonic ischaemia usually occurs at the watershed (Fig. 5.37 ⑩) along the marginal artery ⑦ between the middle colic ④ and left colic branch ⑤ of the inferior mesenteric ② supply to the colon, often as an acute event. Symptoms may include severe abdominal pain, diarrhoea containing dark blood and clots, and systemic upset. There may be a history of atherosclerotic disease elsewhere, and smoking.

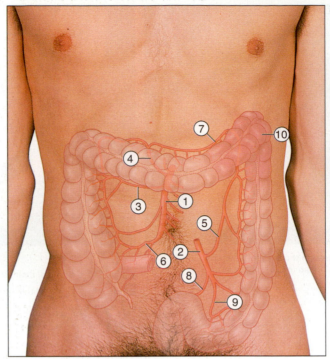

KEY
① Superior mesenteric artery
② Inferior mesenteric artery
③ Right colic artery
④ Middle colic artery
⑤ Left colic artery
⑥ Ileocolic artery
⑦ Marginal artery
⑧ Superior rectal artery
⑨ Sigmoid artery
⑩ Watershed between superior and inferior mesenteric territory

Fig. 5.37 Arterial blood supply to the colon

Examination

On **inspection**, a patient with ischaemic bowel appears pale and clammy, is in pain, has a pyrexia and looks unwell. Abdominal inspection may reveal a distended abdomen, but often the external apparently normal appearance is disproportionate to the severity of the patient's pain. **Palpation** may localize the pain to one part of the abdomen (for colonic ischaemia) or pain may be generalized. Palpation of the radial pulse may identify an irregular beat; emboli from the heart may travel to occlude mesenteric vessels (Fig. 5.37 ①②). **Percussion** will confirm the rebound and guarding. **Auscultation** may be silent as ischaemia then infarction occurs.

Investigation

For acute mesenteric infarction, a high white cell count, acidosis on arterial blood gas analysis and raised amylase strongly support the diagnosis. For less severe ischaemia, a raised white cell count and plasma viscosity may be all that is evident. On plain abdominal radiographs, it may be possible to see radiological changes in the wall of an ischaemic colon (thumbprinting, as if a thumb has pressed on the bowel wall; thickened bowel wall; air in the bowel wall) and a contrast enema may demonstrate the ischaemic colon (Fig. 5.38 ▪1). If chronic ischaemia is suspected, angiography may be useful to indicate which vessels are diseased. Laparoscopy or laparotomy can demonstrate ischaemic small bowel.

Management

Oxygen, analgesia and fluid resuscitation are followed by resection of the ischaemic segment with stoma formation (as an anastomosis will not heal in the presence of ischaemia), unless the full length of intestine is ischaemic, when terminal care is needed.

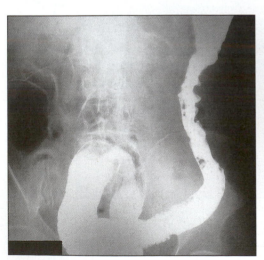

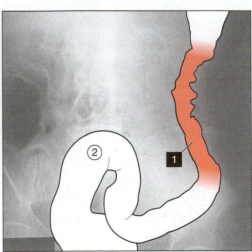

KEY
▪1 Ischaemic descending colon
② Sigmoid colon

Fig. 5.38 Contrast enema of colon showing an ischaemic descending colon

Ovarian mass

The commonest lower abdominal masses are a pregnant uterus (Fig. 5.39 ①) and an enlarged bladder ④ secondary to acute or chronic retention of urine (often in men). One other lower abdominal mass of surgical interest is an ovarian mass due to cyst formation or tumour.

History

For women of potentially childbearing age, ask when the last menstrual period occurred and whether there is any possibility of pregnancy. Acute urinary retention is most common in elderly men who have been experiencing symptoms of bladder outflow obstruction: frequency, nocturia, difficulty in initiating the urinary stream, dribbling at the end of the stream and a poor flow. If an ovarian mass is suspected, lower abdominal discomfort or episodes of more acute lower abdominal pain (related to torsion of the ovarian pedicle Fig. 5.39 ③) may occur; however, even quite large masses (Fig. 5.40) may be asymptomatic until they cause pressure effects on surrounding structures such as the bladder (Fig. 5.39 ④) or bowel (see Bowel obstruction, p. 52) with the accompanying symptoms. A full menstrual history, past history of abdominal surgery, and family history of ovarian, breast or colon cancer is required.

Examination

Look for ascites, cachexia, pallor or jaundice as signs of advanced ovarian malign-ancy. On **inspection** of the abdomen, look for distension, an apparent mass, stretch marks and abdominal scars.

On **palpation**, gently feel for a palpable abdominal mass (Fig. 5.40) and by deeper palpation try to delineate the extent of the mass and whether it arises from the pelvis. **Percussion** can be useful to distinguish a large solid ovarian mass from the surrounding tympanic bowel and to test for the shifting dullness of ascites. Unless the mass is causing obstruction, **auscultation** will be normal.

Investigations

Haematological and biochemical indices may be normal. Tumour markers (CA125, CA153) may be elevated in the presence of an ovarian cancer.

An abdominal ultrasound scan supplemented by CT (Fig. 5.40) or MRI scanning can provide useful diagnostic and staging information. Chest radiology may identify lung or pleural metastases.

Management

Management is by surgical excision or debulking and combination chemotherapy.

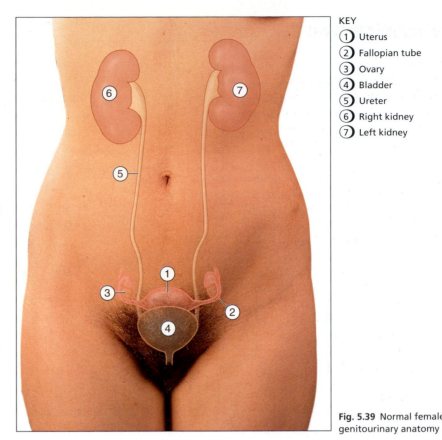

KEY
① Uterus
② Fallopian tube
③ Ovary
④ Bladder
⑤ Ureter
⑥ Right kidney
⑦ Left kidney

Fig. 5.39 Normal female genitourinary anatomy

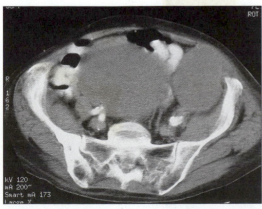

Fig. 5.40 CT scan of pelvis in ovarian cancer

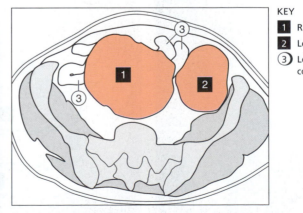

KEY
1 Right ovarian mass
2 Left ovarian mass
3 Loops of bowel containing contrast

BOWEL OBSTRUCTION

In bowel obstruction, a history of colicky waves of abdominal pain may be associated with distension, nausea and vomiting. Borborygmi may be noted by the patient. A history of change in bowel habit, bleeding or mucus per anum should raise the suspicion of bowel cancer or diverticular disease. Medications reducing gut motility (e.g. benzodiazepines, opiates) and electrolyte disturbances (e.g. hypokalaemia postoperatively) need to be remembered.

Bowel obstruction can be classified as due to intraluminal matter (compacted faeces), mechanical obstruction due to thickening of the wall (cancer, inflammatory conditions, post-ischaemia stenosis), extrinsic compression (adhesions), volvulus (sigmoid, caecal) or a pseudo-obstruction from functional motility failure.

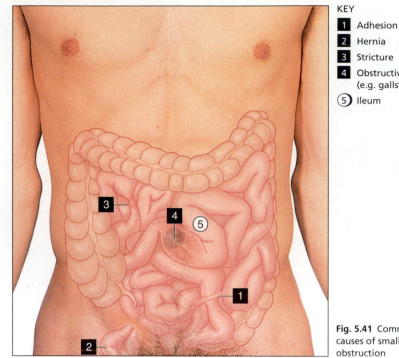

KEY
1 Adhesion
2 Hernia
3 Stricture
4 Obstructive bolus (e.g. gallstone)
5 Ileum

Fig. 5.41 Common causes of small bowel obstruction

Small bowel obstruction

Small bowel obstruction is usually due to adhesions (Fig. 5.41 1), which are commonly secondary to previous surgery but sometimes congenital, small bowel trapped in a hernia 2 , inflammatory conditions of the bowel (such as Crohn's or diverticular disease) causing stricture 3 or bolus obstruction (e.g. a gallstone 'ileus' 4).

History

The history is of gradual onset of waves of abdominal pain described as colicky; there may have been previous episodes over many years. Ask about associated features such as abdominal distension, nausea, vomiting and the content of the vomit (often bile stained or, with more prolonged obstruction distal small bowel content, offensive faeculent vomit). Ask if the patient has noted any particularly tender areas, such as a hernia (Ch. 7) which may be responsible for entrapping the small bowel 2 .

A past history of operations, stoma or fistulae, previous obstructive episodes or ingestion of unusual food stuffs may indicate the cause of the obstruction.

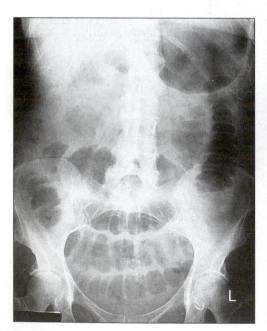

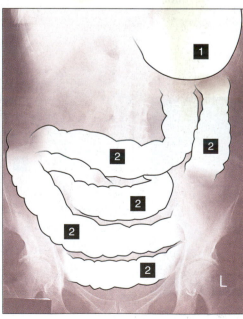

KEY
1 Distended stomach
2 Distended small bowel loops

Fig. 5.42 Plain radiograph of small bowel obstruction

Medications, chronic obstructive pulmonary disease and cardiovascular conditions may either contribute to the obstruction or affect the treament.

Examination
On general physical examination, look for signs of dehydration, and look at the contents of the vomit bowl. **Inspect** the abdomen carefully for surgical scars and herniae, particularly remembering that femoral hernia can be difficult to diagnose. Gentle **palpation** of the abdomen, particularly over any tender areas, may elicit the cause of the bowel obstruction: perhaps a groin hernia or incisional hernia (see Chapter 7).

If there is no obvious external herniation to cause obstruction, superficial then deep palpation of the abdomen will elicit any tenderness or palpable mass.

Percussion will demonstrate a tympanic abdomen and **auscultation** in the early stages of obstruction will reveal active runs of bowel sounds which may be higher pitched than usual. When obstruction persists, and particularly if trapped bowel becomes ischaemic resulting in peritonitis, the abdomen may become silent.

Investigation
Haematology may demonstrate a raised white cell count, ESR/plasma viscosity, and C-reactive protein. With vomiting and progressive dehydration, urea and creatinine will be elevated and sodium, potassium and bicarbonate deranged. Plain radiographs (supine, supplemented by an erect or a decubitus view) will show centrally placed distended loops of small bowel (Fig. 5.42 **2**) and rarely show the cause of the obstruction. Note that the plicae semicircularis (lines across the full diameter of the small bowel) help distinguish small bowel **2** from distended colon (Fig. 5.44).

Management
Oxygen, intravenous fluids and nasogastric aspiration ('drip and suck') may allow the small bowel obstruction to settle spontaneously aided by analgesia. Operative intervention to relieve the obstruction (divide adhesions, remove any necrotic obstructed small bowel, repair any herniation) is required if the small bowel obstruction does not settle rapidly.

Large bowel obstruction

History
In contrast to small bowel obstruction, which is usually due to extrinsic compression, large bowel obstruction (Fig. 5.43 **1**) is usually due to thickening of the wall of the colon – commonly because of colorectal cancer, diverticular disease or inflammatory bowel disease. There is gradual onset of waves of abdominal pain, described as colicky, with abdominal distension and associated nausea and vomiting (initially bile stained or, with more prolonged obstruction, offensive faeculent vomit). There is often a longer history of change in bowel habit (progressive constipation or alternating constipation and diarrhoea), bleeding or mucus per anum, tiredness (due to anaemia) or excessive flatus due to the underlying cause of the large bowel obstruction (see Colorectal cancer, p. 55, Diverticular disease, p. 58, Inflammatory bowel disease, p. 48). A past history of known diverticular disease, previous malignancy (not only intra-abdominal), sigmoid volvulus, or abdominal surgery may point to the underlying cause. Large bowel obstruction can be mimicked by pseudo-obstruction

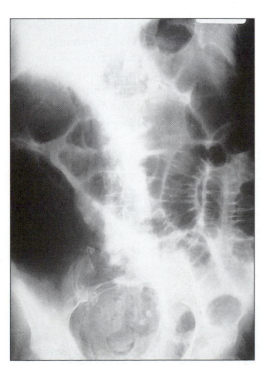
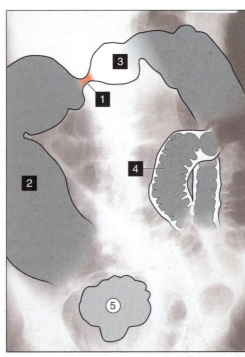

KEY

1 Site of obstruction

2 Distended proximal colon

3 Collapsed transverse colon

4 Loops of small bowel with thickened wall

5 Stool in rectum

Fig. 5.43 Plain abdominal radiograph in transverse colon obstruction

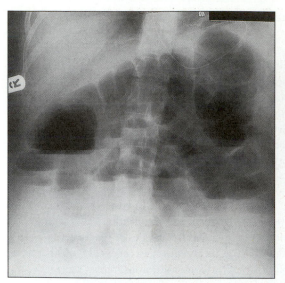
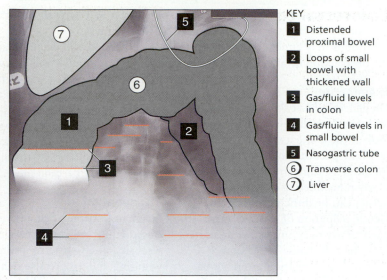

KEY

1 Distended proximal bowel

2 Loops of small bowel with thickened wall

3 Gas/fluid levels in colon

4 Gas/fluid levels in small bowel

5 Nasogastric tube

6 Transverse colon

7 Liver

Fig. 5.44 Erect abdominal radiograph in large bowel obstruction

where the symptoms are remarkably similar to true obstruction, but due to medications, electrolyte derangements, immobility or a combination of all three. Thus a drug and social history is important. Cardiorespiratory co-morbidity can significantly influence symptoms and treatment options.

Examination

On general physical examination, look for signs of dehydration, and look at the contents of the vomit bowl. **Inspect** the abdomen carefully for surgical scars, distension, asymmetry and masses. Gentle **palpation** of the abdomen, particularly over any tender areas, may elicit the cause of the bowel obstruction: deeper palpation may delineate the presence of a mass causing the obstruction.

Rectal examination (at which time rigid sigmoidoscopy may be performed) is required to identify any obstructing rectal lesion.

Percussion will demonstrate a distended tympanic abdomen.

Auscultation will demonstrate active runs of high pitched bowel sounds. With long-standing obstruction, particularly if accompanied by perforation of the distended bowel resulting in peritonitis, the abdomen becomes silent.

Investigation

Haematology may demonstrate microcytic anaemia (due to chronic blood loss), a raised white cell count, ESR/plasma viscosity, and C-reactive protein. With vomiting and progressive dehydration, urea and creatinine may be elevated and sodium, potassium and bicarbonate deranged. Plain supine radiographs (Fig. 5.43), will show distended colon down to **2** but not beyond **3** the level of the obstruction **1**. In addition, on an erect (Fig. 5.44) or a decubitus view, centrally placed distended loops of small bowel are commonly identified **2** and air/fluid levels **3** **4** may be seen. A contrast enema per anum should identify the site of the obstruction, and will at least exclude pseudo-obstruction. Colonoscopy in skilled hands may also identify the site and cause of the obstruction, and CT can be used to provide additional information.

Management

Oxygen (the distended abdomen often compromises respiratory activity), intravenous fluids, and nasogastric aspiration Fig. 5.44 **5** ('drip and suck') are used for resuscitation. Most causes of large bowel obstruction require operative intervention – in the emergency situa-tion, excision of the obstructing lesion is performed, usually with formation of a stoma (see page 60), but oc-casionally with primary anastomosis. Alternatively, a defunctioning stoma may relieve the obstruction and allow an elective operation.

Colorectal cancer

Colorectal cancer is common and reflects the low fibre western diet. The presenting complaints can be non-specific and may cause diagnostic confusion with diverticular disease, irritable bowel syndrome or haemorrhoids.

History

When taking a history, ask about vague lower abdominal discomfort and bloatedness, which are common. The classic symptoms are fresh bleeding on or mixed in with the the stool (for rectal/sigmoid carcinoma), change in bowel habit (constipation or loose, frequent stools), or symptoms of anaemia (breathlessness, tiredness) secondary to blood loss (from right side colon or caecal cancer). Rectal cancers (and adenomas) may produce considerable mucus. Rectal cancers may also give a feeling of urgency (tenesmus) or incomplete emptying and, if locally advanced, may cause perineal pain or involve the sphincters to result in faecal incontinence.

A family history of colon cancer (particularly first degree relatives under the age of 45), polyposis or a past history of polyps, ulcerative colitis or Crohn's disease increases the risk of developing colorectal cancer. A second (metachronous) carcinoma occurs in some 5% of individuals, so ask about any previous history of colorectal cancer.

The patient may have been taking medication to relieve constipation and iron (causing black stools) to improve anaemia.

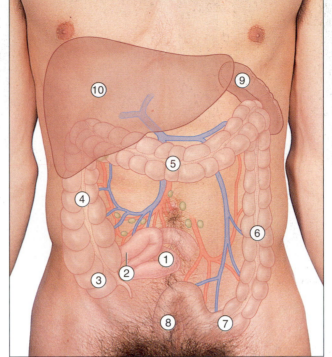

KEY
1. Ileum
2. Terminal ileum
3. Caecum
4. Ascending colon
5. Transverse colon
6. Descending colon
7. Sigmoid colon
8. Rectum
9. Spleen
10. Liver

Fig. 5.45 Normal anatomy of large bowel

Examination

Look for general signs of gastrointestinal disease or malignancy. Weight loss, jaundice (secondary to liver metastases) and debility are late signs of advanced disease. Pallor or leuconychia secondary to anaemia may be evident.

On **inspection** of the abdomen, there may be no outward sign of the carcinoma within. In thin individuals with a large lesion, a mass may be visible, or the backlog of faeces behind a progressively obstructing colonic carcinoma may be evident as a mass. An obstructing carcinoma may present signs of large bowel obstruction (see p. 53). A grossly enlarged liver secondary to liver metastases (see p. 40) may be visible in a cachectic individual.

On **palpation**, gentle palpation followed by deeper palpation of the abdomen may delineate a palpable colonic mass (Fig. 5.46 **1**); it should be possible to indent a faecal mass, whereas a palpable cancer is solid but may be mobile (given the mesentery, for example, of the sigmoid colon). The size, position and fixity of the mass can be described.

Rectal (per anal) examination, traditionally with the patient in the left lateral position, knees curled up, is crucial to identifying the presence of a lesion in the rectum. If a lump or mass

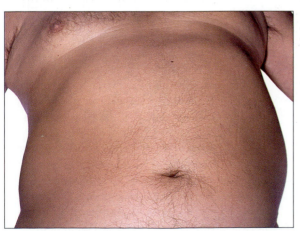

Fig. 5.46 Caecal carcinoma

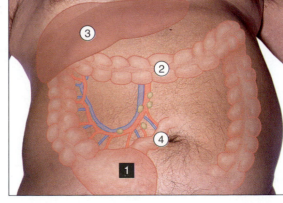

KEY
1 Caecal carcinoma
2. Colon
3. Liver
4. Ileum

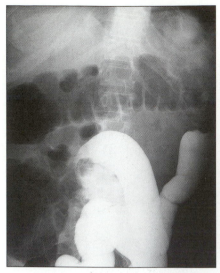

Fig. 5.47 Synchronous carcinomas of colon

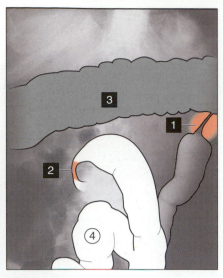

KEY

1. Splenic flexure carcinoma
2. Sigmoid carcinoma
3. Dilated transverse colon
4. Normal sigmoid colon

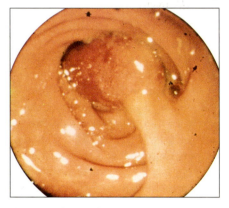

Fig. 5.48 Polyp in colon

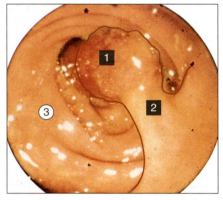

KEY

1. Bleeding polyp
2. Stalk
3. Normal colon

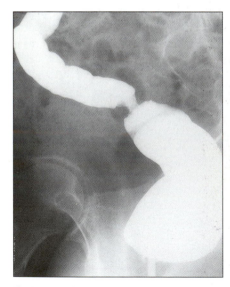

Fig. 5.49 Single contrast barium enema of rectosigmoid cancer

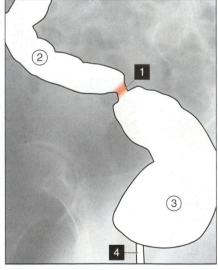

KEY

1. Applecore deformity, rectosigmoid junction
2. Sigmoid colon
3. Rectum
4. Tube to instil contrast

is palpable, it is important to describe its position (anterior, posterior, lateral), distance from the anorectal junction (which may dictate whether the anus can be preserved during surgery for a cancer), size/extent, mobility (e.g. highly mobile like a polyp, Fig. 5.48) or fixity (e.g. a rectal carcinoma invading the sacral tissues), and the involvement of other structures (such as the vagina). If the rectal mucosa feels normal, a sample of stool, if present, can be removed on the gloved digit to test for faecal occult blood, which may be the only indication on clinical examination of a polyp or carcinoma lurking proximally in the colon.

Percussion can be used to assess whether an abdominal mass is apparently more solid (Fig. 5.46 **1**) than the surrounding tympanic normal bowel. Percussion for shifting dullness can also be used to look for ascites. **Auscultation** may be normal in a patient with colorectal carcinoma, although if the cancer obstructs the bowel, sounds may become obstructive.

Investigation

A full blood count should look for microcytic anaemia from blood loss into the colon. Plasma viscosity/ESR may be raised. Urea and creatinine may be elevated in advanced cancer of the rectum (owing to ureteric obstruction) and abnormal LFTs may signify liver metastases. A grossly raised carcino-embryonic antigen (CEA) may also suggest the presence of metastases.

A plain radiograph of the chest and an ultrasound scan of the liver should be used to seek metastatic disease. A contrast enhanced CT scan or MRI scan may be used to look for liver metastases and assess local invasion by a rectal cancer.

Prior to surgery on the colon or rectum, all of the large bowel needs to be imaged for synchronous second cancers (Fig. 5.47 **1** **2**) or polyps (Fig. 5.48 **1**). In the clinic, rigid sigmoidoscopy and proctoscopy can supplement rectal examination to visualize, assess invasion using endoscopic ultrasound, and biopsy a rectal cancer. Barium enema examination (single contrast, Fig. 5.49 or double contrast using contrast plus air) can outline the remaining colon to the terminal ileum, provided the

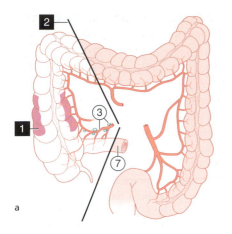
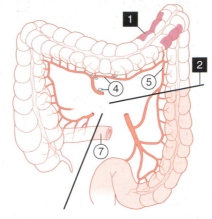
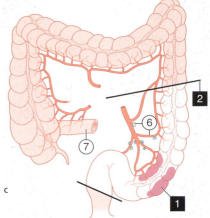

Fig. 5.50 Surgical resection: (**a**) right hemicolectomy, (**b**) extended right hemicolectomy, (**c**) anterior resection. Healthy (pink) bowel can be anastomosed after resection of the cancer

KEY

1 Cancer
2 Extent of resection
3 Ileocolic artery and nodes
4 Middle colic artery and nodes
5 Marginal artery
6 Inferior mesenteric artery and nodes
7 Ileum

bowel is adequately cleared first (usually using oral purgative solutions), although colonoscopy in experienced hands may have the advantage of allowing biopsy of any visible abnormalities. In some centres, a combination of barium enema and flexible sigmoidoscopy is used to ensure that the sigmoid colon (which has a high incidence of cancers, Figs 5.47 and 5.49, and is more difficult to visualize on barium enema) is adequately examined.

Treatment

The mainstay of treatment is surgical resection of the cancer (Fig. 5.51) together with the draining lymph nodes and is based on the anatomical blood supply of the colon (Figs 5.50 a, b, c) such that any anastomosis has the greatest chance of healing. For rectal cancers, mesorectal excision of the tissues around the rectum is required to get clearance around the cancer. Under circumstances where an anastomosis is ill-advised (emergency surgery) or impossible (an abdomino-perineal resection of the rectum), a colostomy or ileostomy will be necessary (p. 60). On the basis of Dukes' staging (Table 5.6) and TNM staging, further, adjuvant therapy may be given. Post-operative chemotherapy for Dukes' C cancers and preoperative or postoperative radiotherapy for rectal cancer can be used as additional therapy to reduce the chances of systemic and local disease recurrence respectively.

Table 5.6 Dukes' classification	
Dukes' A	Cancer confined to colon wall
Dukes' B	Cancer penetrating colon wall
Dukes' C_1	Involving mesenteric lymph nodes
C_2	Most proximal node (in resection specimen) involved with tumour
Dukes' D	Distant (liver) metastases*
* Dukes' D is used clinically but was not orginally described by Cuthbert Dukes.	

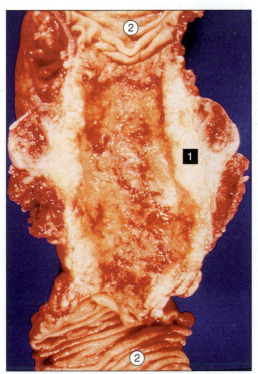

KEY

1 Colon cancer
2 Normal colon

Fig. 5.51 Colon carcinoma

Diverticular disease

Diverticular disease (Fig. 5.52), like colorectal cancer, is increasingly common with age and reflects the low fibre western diet. Inflammation of one or more diverticula, a process known as diverticulitis (Fig. 5.53 **3**), may cause marked symptoms, although many people with uncomplicated diverticular disease are asymptomatic. The presenting complaints can be non-specific and may cause diagnostic confusion with colorectal cancer, inflammatory bowel disease or irritable bowel syndrome.

History

In the history, ask about lower abdominal discomfort and bloatedness, which are common. Constipation, pelleted stools, offensive flatus, mucus per anum and blood mixed in with the stool are symptoms strongly associated with diverticular disease. On occasion, diverticular disease may present with a brisk fresh rectal bleed (Fig. 5.53 **5**) from the neck of a diverticulum, which is alarming to the patient but usually self limiting. These are also classic symptoms of colorectal cancer and both conditions may occur in the same individual; hence even in the presence of known diverticular disease, any new symptoms should be investigated to exclude the recent development of a colorectal cancer. Fistulation from a diverticulum to the bladder **6** (resulting in symptoms of frequent urinary tract infection due to gut organisms which recurs despite adequate antibiotic treatment, or even pneumaturia), to another part of the bowel, to the vagina (particularly in a woman who has had a hysterectomy; resulting in a brown offensive vaginal discharge) may cause symptoms. Local abscess **7** formation may result in complaints of localized tenderness and fever.

The patient may have been taking medication to relieve the constipation caused by the thickened walls and narrowed lumen **4** of a colon affected by diverticular disease.

Examination

On examination, there may be signs of systemic upset (fever) or blood loss (pallor) due to complications of diverticular disease. However, most patients show few systemic signs on presentation.

On **inspection** of the abdomen, a diverticular mass may be visible in the left iliac fossa, secondary to local inflammation **3** or abscess **7** formation. On **palpation**, gentle superficial then deep palpation of the abdomen may delineate a palpable sigmoid colon, the bowel most frequently involved in diverticular disease. On rectal examination, a tender diverticular mass may be palpable on the left side, although the rectal wall should feel normal. A stool specimen should be tested for faecal occult blood. Vaginal examination with a speculum will be appropriate if there is a history of vaginal discharge suggestive of a fistula.

Percussion can be used to assess whether an abdominal mass is solid relative to the surrounding tympanic normal bowel. Following perforation (Fig. 5.53 **1**) large amounts of free peritoneal air (Fig. 5.54 **1**) may make the abdomen tympanic. **Auscultation** should be normal unless the diverticular disease causes bowel obstruction (Fig. 5.53 **4**) or peritonitis secondary to perforation **1** **2** .

Investigation

Urine testing should be used to look for evidence of urinary infection.

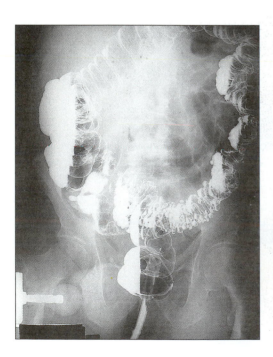
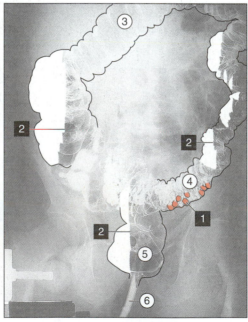

KEY

1	Diverticulae
2	Contrast level
③	Transverse colon
④	Sigmoid colon
⑤	Rectum
⑥	Rectal catheter

Fig. 5.52 Double contrast enema demonstrating diverticular disease (radiographs taken with the patient lying on his side)

Blood tests include a full blood count and measurement of plasma viscosity, looking for microcytic anaemia from blood loss into the colon and a raised white cell count and plasma viscosity secondary to inflammation. Plain abdominal and erect chest (Fig. 5.54) films may demonstrate free intraperitoneal air **1**. An ultrasound scan, CT scan or MRI scan of the abdomen may demonstrate a diverticular mass. In the absence of acute symptoms, rigid or flexible sigmoidoscopy combined with contrast enema examination (usually double contrast with barium plus air, Fig. 5.52) can outline the diseased bowel and ensure that the sigmoid colon is adequately visualized.

Management

Symptom control using dietary manipulation and antispasmodics, antibiotics for episodes of inflammation and careful observation and intravenous support at the time of acute, self-limiting bleeding mean that colonic resection is required only for complications of diverticular disease (Fig. 5.53): perforation **1**, obstruction **4**, fistulation **6**, abscess formation **7** and major haemorrhage **5**.

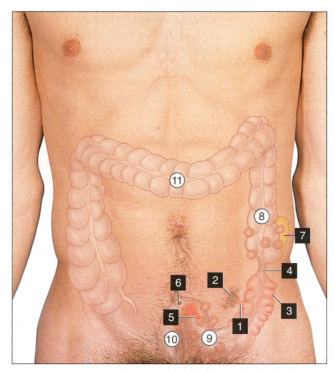

Fig. 5.53 Complications of diverticular disease

KEY

1 Perforation	**6** Fistula – to bladder (bladder not shown)
2 Gas, faeces, etc from perforation	**7** Abscess
3 Acute inflammation	⑧ Descending colon
4 Thick wall, narrow lumen stricture	⑨ Sigmoid colon
5 Bleeding	⑩ Rectum
	⑪ Transverse colon

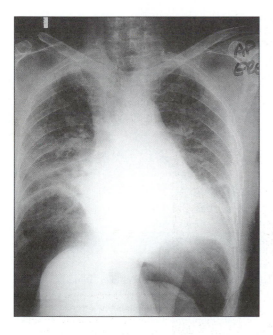

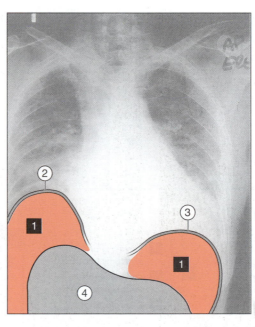

KEY

① Free intraperitoneal air
② Right hemidiaphragm
③ Left hemidiaphragm
④ Liver

Fig. 5.54 Erect chest radiograph following perforated sigmoid colon

Stoma

History

A stoma, or opening of the bowel onto the abdominal wall, is used to discharge bowel or urinary contents into a bag, where discontinuity of the gastrointestinal or urinary tracts is necessary. Ask the patient why, when and under what circumstances the stoma (or stomata if there are more than one) was formed. What sort of fluid or solid comes out? Is the stoma permanent or temporary and, if there is more than one, which one is productive? A past surgical and medical history is important. Dietary restrictions, excessive fluid loss, and any bleeding or mucus from the stoma may indicate dysfunction.

Examination

On **inspection** (Figs 5.55 and 5.56), look at the site(s) of the stoma **1** **2**, identify the sites of the surgical scars **3** and from an understanding of the type of stoma (Fig. 5.57, Table 5.7) and the underlying anatomy, determine what the stoma does. **Palpation** should include, for a gastrointestinal tract stoma, gloved digital examination to ensure there is no obstruction or stricture of the stoma. **Percussion** or **auscultation** is helpful if bowel obstruction is suspected.

Investigation

Contrast enema or endoscopy through the stoma provides useful examination of the bowel just upstream or downstream from the stoma if bleeding from or obstruction of the stoma occurs.

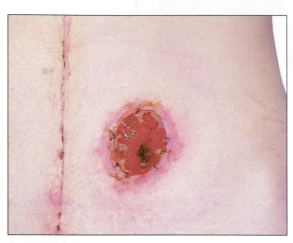

Fig. 5.55 End colostomy

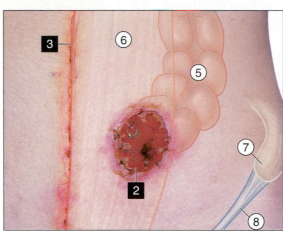

KEY

1	Ileostomy
2	Colostomy
3	Laparotomy scar
4	Intra-abdominal ileum
5	Descending colon
6	Rectus sheath
7	Anterior superior iliac spine
8	Inguinal ligament

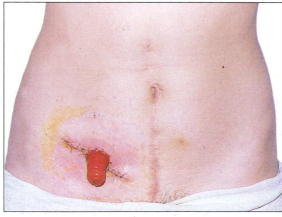

Fig. 5.56 Ileostomy

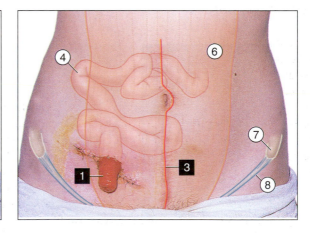

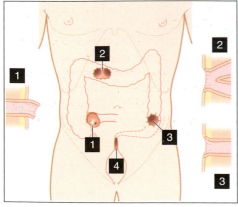

Fig. 5.57 Abdominal stoma

KEY

1	Ileostomy or urostomy (spout)
2	Double-barrel (loop) colostomy
3	End colostomy
4	Mucous fistula

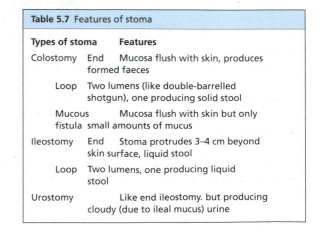

Table 5.7 Features of stoma

Types of stoma		Features
Colostomy	End	Mucosa flush with skin, produces formed faeces
	Loop	Two lumens (like double-barrelled shotgun), one producing solid stool
	Mucous fistula	Mucosa flush with skin but only small amounts of mucus
Ileostomy	End	Stoma protrudes 3–4 cm beyond skin surface, liquid stool
	Loop	Two lumens, one producing liquid stool
Urostomy		Like end ileostomy. but producing cloudy (due to ileal mucus) urine

6 Perineum

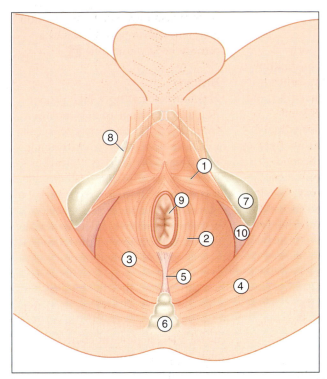

Fig. 6.1 Normal anatomy of the perineum

KEY
1. Transversus perinei superficialis
2. Sphincter ani externus
3. Levator ani
4. Gluteus maximus
5. Anococcygeal ligament
6. Coccyx
7. Ischial tuberosity
8. Inferior pubic ramus
9. Anus
10. Ischiorectal fossa

History

The age and sex of the patient are important: perianal sepsis tends to occur in young and middle-aged males (although it certainly occurs in females), haemorrhoids in older people and in pregnant women.

Ask about the onset of symptoms, the presence of tenderness and pain in the perineum and perianal area: does pain occur on defaecation only (suggestive of a fissure), or is there persistent pain (if so for how long)? Is there any bleeding – red or dark blood – and what is the timing in relation to defaecation? Haemorrhoids are associated with fresh red blood on toilet paper or underwear, a fissure with painful defaecation and fresh red blood on the stool, and colorectal cancer by blood mixed in with the stool. Is there any mucous discharge (which may be associated with haemorrhoids)? Constipation may be associated with development of a perianal fissure or abscess; alternatively, irregular bowel habit or diarrhoea may be associated with underlying inflammatory bowel disease or colorectal cancer.

The past history may include previous episodes of perianal sepsis or haemorrhoids, surgical drainage of an abscess, or operative procedures on haemorrhoids. Traumatic childbirth may cause disruption of the perineum. Medications, particularly opioids, may cause constipation and be associated with perianal sepsis.

The general history should include concurrent medical conditions such as diabetes, as anaesthesia is often required to fully assess and treat perineal problems.

Examination

Look for systemic signs of sepsis (with associated pyrexia); smell the patient's breath for the fetor of constipation. Does the patient sit comfortably or prefer to lie on one side or stand? The perineum may be too tender to perform a detailed examination without anaesthesia. However, with the patient in the left lateral position, with hips flexed, it should be possible to inspect for signs of sepsis or prolapsed haemorrhoids by parting the buttocks. Under general or regional anaesthesia, more detailed inspection and palpation, including rectal examination, proctoscopy and sigmoidoscopy (rigid or flexible), will demonstrate the pathological process and facilitate treatment.

Investigation

Urine and blood should be tested for diabetes. The white cell count may be raised (with a neutrophilia) in the presence of perineal sepsis; other routine blood tests, chest radiograph and ECG may be required as part of the anaesthetic work-up.

Any pus obtained at surgery from a perianal abscess should be Gram stained and cultured – gastrointestinal organisms suggest an origin in the GI tract, whereas staphylococcal organisms suggest a skin origin. For recurrent sepsis, part of the abscess cavity should be excised and sent for pathology examination to exclude Crohn's disease.

Once the acute episode has been treated, bowel investigations (colonoscopy or barium enema with sigmoidoscopy) may be required to exclude concomitant colorectal cancer or underlying inflammatory bowel disease.

Haemorrhoids

Haemorrhoids remain poorly understood but it is helpful to know a classification for communication with colleagues. First-degree haemorrhoids (Fig. 6.2 **1**) are not visible on inspection of the anus, nor palpable on digital rectal examination, but can be seen on proctoscopy. Second-degree haemorrhoids **2** prolapse though the anal margin but spontaneously return into the anal canal. Third-degree haemorrhoids have prolapsed **3** but will return into the anal canal with manipulation. A fourth-degree haemorrhoid cannot be replaced into the anal canal and may be thrombosed (Fig. 6.3 **1**). Haemorrhoids originating from the anorectal mucosa are sometimes known as internal haemorrhoids or piles (Fig. 6.2 **1** **2** **3**), and a perianal haematoma at the anal–skin margin is confusingly known as a thrombosed external pile **4** .

History

Haemorrhoids afflict a high proportion of the western adult population from time to time and may reflect the low fibre western diet and straining on defaecation. There is typically a history of constipation, anal discomfort (rather than pain), red spotting of blood on toilet paper and mucous staining of underwear. There may be episodes of prolapse of the haemorrhoids, spontaneously returning, requiring manual replacement (Fig. 6.3 **2**), or thrombosing **1** with subsequent fibrosis to form anal skin tags **3** . Most patients know the diagnosis, but concomitant colorectal or anal neoplasia must be excluded. The history should include past episodes of perianal symptoms and any previous surgery.

Examination

With the patient in the left lateral position, parting the buttocks will demonstrate prolapsed haemorrhoids, anal skin tags (from resolved haemorrhoids) and any additional perianal pathology. First-degree haemorrhoids are not visible, but look at the position of the skin tags (Fig. 6.3 **3**) and visible haemorrhoids **2** , described as if looking at the face of a clock (12 o'clock position anterior) with the classic positions being at 4, 7 and 11 o'clock. Thrombosed, purple, oedematous haemorrhoids **1** are painful.

Treatment

Haemorrhoids, even acutely prolapsed haemorrhoids (Fig. 6.3 **1**), will resolve and fibrose to form skin tags **3** over several days. Bed rest, analgesia (non-constipating), a stool softener, local application of ice packs or lignocaine gel ease discomfort while resolution occurs. First- and second-degree haemorrhoids may be successfully treated by banding, injecting sclerosant at the base of the haemorrhoid or infra-red coagulation where dietary measures alone have failed. Surgical excision or stapling is usually reserved for second- or third-degree haemorrhoids.

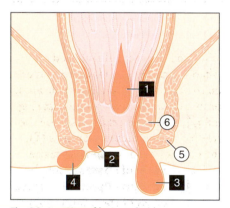

KEY

1 First degree haemorrhoid
2 Second degree haemorrhoid
3 Third degree haemorrhoid
4 Perianal haematoma ('external pile')
⑤ External sphincter
⑥ Internal sphincter

Fig. 6.2 Anatomy of haemorrhoids

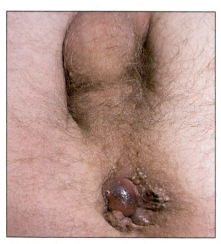

Fig. 6.3 Haemorrhoids

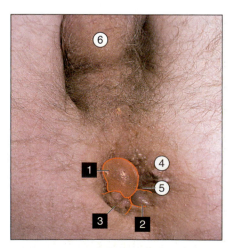

KEY

1 Haemorrhoid at 11 o'clock
2 Haemorrhoid at 4 o'clock
3 Skin tag at 7 o'clock
④ Anus
⑤ Anal orifice
⑥ Scrotum

Anal fissure

History

The classic history is for a (usually) young person to experience sharp pain on defaecation (described as like passing glass per anum) with an associated small amount of fresh blood on the stool and toilet paper. There is usually a history of constipation, and the problem may be intermittent as the anal mucosa heals over and then tears again.

Examination

Inspection of the anus demonstrates the fissure (Fig. 6.4 **1**) classically in the 6 o'clock position, although less commonly it may lie at any other position of the imaginary clock face. By gentle distraction of the anus, the fissure can be seen, often with a sentinel tag **2** at the external end, and the internal sphincter fibres **3** may be visible in the base of the fissure.

Treatment

Treatment can be by local application of glycerine trinitrate cream and dietary modification (to improve the bulk of the stool and reduce constipation), failing which surgical incision of the internal sphincter (lateral sphincterotomy) under anaesthetic will stop the painful spasm.

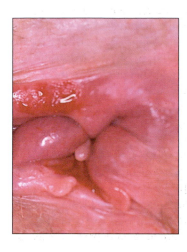
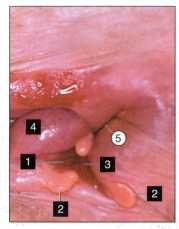

KEY

1 Fissure
2 Sentinel tags
3 Internal sphincter
4 Haemorrhoid
(5) Anal orifice

Fig. 6.4 Anal fissure and haemorrhoid

Perineal sepsis

History

Increasing dull continuous throbbing pain in the perineum or perianal region, often worse on defaecation (hence the patient becomes constipated) and usually too painful to sit normally, are the prominent symptoms. Usually occurring in young men, repeat episodes suggest an underlying fistula from the anorectal mucosa or inflammatory bowel disease (Crohn's). Ischiorectal abscess (Fig. 6.5 **1**) and perianal abscess **4** are most common; perineal skin sepsis (e.g. in a sebaceous cyst), intersphincteric **3** abscess and suprasphincteric **2** abscesses are less common.

Examination

The anatomy of the perineum and lower gastrointestinal tract (Figs 6.1 and 6.5) is the key to understanding what one can see and feel. Find out whether the signs of inflammation are on the left or right side, on both sides, or in continuity; look for redness (Fig. 6.6 **1**), swelling, tenderness, and the relationship of these to the anus (3), the muscles of the region and hence deduce the type of abscess. Look for scars **2** and signs of previous surgery, and the redness of spreading cellulitis. From the position of the most

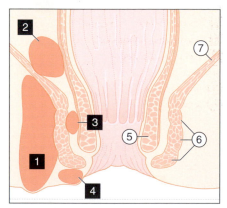

Fig. 6.5 Anatomy of anorectal abscess sites

KEY

1 Ischiorectal abscess
2 Suprasphincteric abscess
3 Intersphincteric abscess
4 Perianal abscess
(5) Internal sphincter
(6) External sphincter
(7) Levator ani

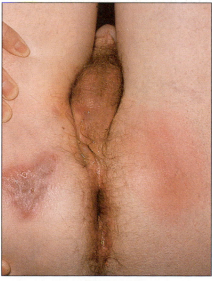

Fig. 6.6 Perineal sepsis   KEY

1 Ischiorectal abscess
2 Scar from previous ischiorectal abscess

(3) Anus
(4) Scrotum

inflamed skin and if the abscess is pointing, it should be possible to decide whether the abscess is ischiorectal (Fig. 6.6 **1**) or perianal. Palpation and rectal examination are usually too painful without anaesthesia. Under anaesthesia, the indurated tissues around the abscess can be palpated, with attention to any intersphincteric abscess (Fig. 6.5 **3**) felt in the wall of the anal canal or suprasphincteric abscess **2** palpable through the lower rectal wall.

Proctoscopy and sigmoidoscopy rarely show the (presumed) originally intraluminal origin of the abscess but allow examination and, if abnormal, biopsy of the rectal mucosa.

Investigation

Apart from a full blood count to demonstrate a raised white cell count, Gram stain, culture and sensitivity of the pus and biopsy of the abscess wall (for recurrent sepsis) are the most useful tests. MRI or transanal

ultrasound may be useful in detecting complex sepsis or underlying fistulae after an acute episode.

Treatment

Treatment is by incision and drainage under general or regional anaesthesia with pus sent for bacteriological examination. Subsequent examination under anaesthesia may reveal the presence of fistulae, which may be quite complex, underlying the abscess.

Fistula

A fistula (communication between two epithelial-lined surfaces) opening onto the perineum usually has its origin in the anal canal (Fig. 6.7). A fistula may be simple (passing directly from the anal mucosa to the perineal skin **1**) or complex (passing between the two epithelial surfaces through the sphincteric muscles **2**, branching and having multiple openings).

History

Sometimes following on from a previous history of one or recurrent abscesses in the perineal region, the young (usually) person will complain of a persistent, intermittent purulent discharge (Fig. 6.8 **1**) in the perineum. Unusually, flatus may pass out through the fistula tract. There may be local tenderness or occasional bleeding from the granulation tissue at the external opening **1**. Inflammatory bowel disease should be excluded. Ask for a full medical and surgical history including operations and problems in the perineum; ask about the full range of gastrointestinal symptoms, particularly weight loss, abdominal symptoms, diarrhoea (with or without mucus and blood), and any family history of Crohn's disease.

Examination

On inspection, one or more external openings of the fistula (Fig. 6.8 **1**) may be apparent and may be some distance from the anal margin. There may be granulation tissue at the

external opening, pus **1** or blood. On digital rectal examination, proctoscopy and sigmoidoscopy, an internal opening to the fistula may be visible and palpable.

Investigations

MRI or transanal ultrasound may be useful in detecting simple or complex fistulae, anatomical disruption of the sphincters after an acute episode of sepsis or if there is a chronic problem.

Treatment

Simple fistulae are treated either by laying them open or by excision; complex and high fistulae **2** require expert attention to avoid damaging the complex sphincter mechanisms.

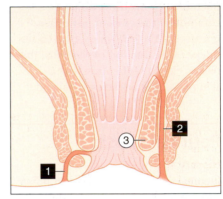

Fig. 6.7 Anatomy of anorectal fistulae

KEY

1 Superficial fistula
2 High fistula
③ Internal sphincter
④ Anus
⑤ Anal orifice

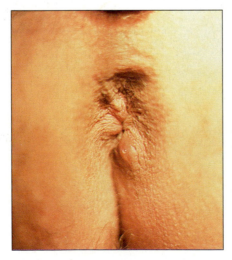

Fig. 6.8 Fistula

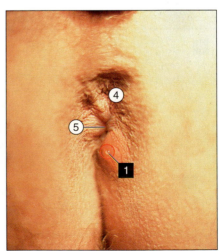

7 Hernia

A hernia can be defined as the abnormal protrusion of an organ or tissues outside their normal body cavity or constraining sheath.

The normal anatomy of the abdominal wall and groin (Fig. 7.1) has several potential weak spots where fascia planes meet, e.g. linea alba ⑧, or structures penetrate the abdominal wall, e.g. spermatic cord ⑦, passing through the deep inguinal ring ⑨ along the inguinal canal and out through the superficial inguinal ring ③.

Abdominal wall hernias occur through points of congenital weakness or through surgical scars (incisional hernia (Fig. 7.2 **5**). Groin hernias occur at the weak points of the inguinal canal (indirect **10** and direct **7** inguinal hernias) or femoral canal (femoral hernias **9**).

Abdominal hernias may contain a range of intra-abdominal structures. These may include:

- Omentum
- Bowel (small bowel, colon)
- Bladder/colon (in sliding hernia)
- Appendix
- Meckel's diverticulum (in Littré's hernia)
- Ovary/fallopian tube

The contents of a hernia are held within a sac (Fig. 7.3a) but it is the neck of the sac which when narrow results in an irreducible (Fig. 7.3b), obstructed (Fig.7.3c) or strangulated (Fig. 7.3d) hernia.

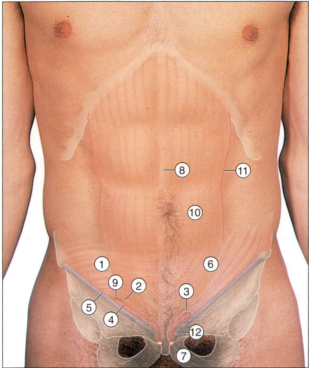

KEY

① Internal oblique
② Conjoint tendon
③ Superficial inguinal ring
④ Cremaster muscle
⑤ Inguinal ligament
⑥ Aponeurosis of external oblique
⑦ Spermatic cord
⑧ Linea alba
⑨ Deep inguinal ring
⑩ Rectus muscle
⑪ Rectus sheath
⑫ Pubic tubercle

Fig. 7.1 Normal anatomy of the lower abdominal wall

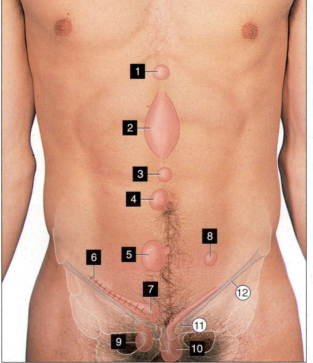

KEY

1 Epigastric
2 Divarication of the recti
3 Paraumbilical
4 Umbilical
5 Incisional
6 Previous hernia repair scar
7 Direct inguinal
8 Spigelian
9 Femoral
10 Indirect inguinal
⑪ Pubic tubercle
⑫ Inguinal ligament

Fig. 7.2 Location of hernias

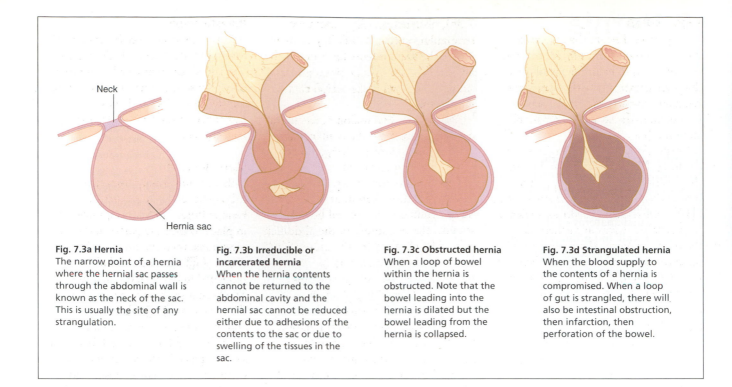

Fig. 7.3a Hernia
The narrow point of a hernia where the hernial sac passes through the abdominal wall is known as the neck of the sac. This is usually the site of any strangulation.

Fig. 7.3b Irreducible or incarcerated hernia
When the hernia contents cannot be returned to the abdominal cavity and the hernial sac cannot be reduced either due to adhesions of the contents to the sac or due to swelling of the tissues in the sac.

Fig. 7.3c Obstructed hernia
When a loop of bowel within the hernia is obstructed. Note that the bowel leading into the hernia is dilated but the bowel leading from the hernia is collapsed.

Fig. 7.3d Strangulated hernia
When the blood supply to the contents of a hernia is compromised. When a loop of gut is strangled, there will also be intestinal obstruction, then infarction, then perforation of the bowel.

Abdominal wall hernias

History

Ask about the position (Fig. 7.2) and duration of the swelling, any discomfort, tenderness or redness of the hernia. Does the swelling disappear when lying flat or can the swelling be manipulated back (reduced) through the abdominal wall with the muscles relaxed? Have there been previous symptomatic episodes? Is any tenderness associated with symptoms of obstruction (abdominal swelling, nausea, vomiting, abdominal pain). Ask about previous abdominal surgery (Fig. 7.4 **2**), whether the hernia is related to a scar (Fig. 7.4 **1**), and whether there were wound complications (infection, dehiscence) postoperatively. Ask about predisposing factors such as lifting heavy weights, chronic cough, constipation or symptoms of bladder outflow obstruction. A general medical history is required prior to surgical treatment of the hernia to ascertain fitness for surgery.

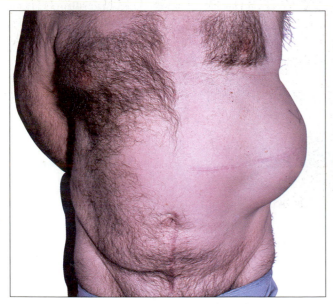

Fig. 7.4 Incisional hernia

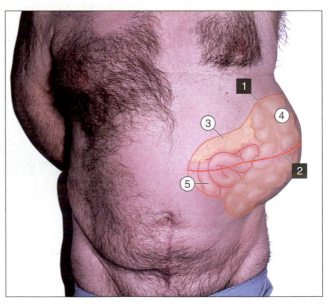

KEY

1 Extent of hernia
2 Surgical scar
③ Omentum
④ Colon
⑤ Jejunum

Examination

Exposure. Ensure that the abdomen is exposed from nipples to groin to allow you to examine for all possible sites of hernias with the patient lying comfortably. Some hernias are best demonstrated with the patient standing (Fig. 7.4).

Inspection. Look for obvious swellings **1** and scars **2** and relate the position, size and shape of the hernia (Fig. 7.5) to the anatomy ③ ④ ⑤. Observe any redness, oedema or peristaltic waves in the hernia. In the obese or where there are multiple operative scars this can be challenging. Ask the patient to cough, protruding any hernia. Ask the patient to manipulate (reduce) the hernia back inside the abdomen if this is possible. Also look for signs of dehydration (dry tongue, flaccid skin) if the patient has been vomiting.

Palpation. Ask if the hernia is tender or sore before feeling the neck of the hernia sac; a wide neck (Fig. 7.4 **1**) is less dangerous than a tight neck (Fig. 7.3a) which will entrap the sac contents, leading to incarceration (Fig. 7.3b), obstruction (Fig. 7.3c) then strangulation (Fig. 7.3d). Try to manipulate the sac contents back inside the abdomen – bowel may give a gurgling sound – but stop if the action elicits tenderness.

Percussion. Percussion of the hernia may be tympanic if the contents are air-containing intestine (Fig. 7.4 ④ ⑤), or appear to be solid if omentum ③ or fluid predominates.

Auscultation. Auscultation of the hernia contents may reveal bowel sounds; the remainder of the abdomen should be checked for the presence of bowel sounds, which may be increased (because of obstruction within the hernia, Fig. 7.3c) or reduced/absent if peritonitis has occurred secondary to strangulation (Fig. 7.3d). Note that a pantaloon hernia (Fig. 7.13) sliding hernia, Richter's hernia, Maydl's hernia and Littré's hernia are rare variations of abdominal wall and groin hernias (see Fig. 7.14).

Investigations

All investigations may be normal in an asymptomatic hernia. If tissues are entrapped, the white cell count and plasma viscosity may increase. Urea, electrolytes, ECG and chest radiograph may be useful prior to anaesthesia.

Management

If there is intestinal obstruction following rehydration using intravenous fluids, and a nasogastric tube in place to aspirate gastro-intestinal secretions, then the previous incision (Fig. 7.4 **2**) can be carefully reopened under general anaesthesia. The hernia sac can be exposed, and the contents ③ ④ ⑤, dissected free and examined to ensure that no strangulation has occurred, before the sac is replaced into the abdomen. The wound is then securely resutured. Reinforcement with a mesh may be required. For other abdominal wall hernias (e.g. Figs 7.5 and 7.6) the sac **1** should similarly be dissected free and the, usually small, defect **2** closed with non-absorbable sutures.

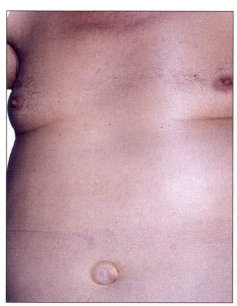

Fig. 7.5 Paraumbilical hernia

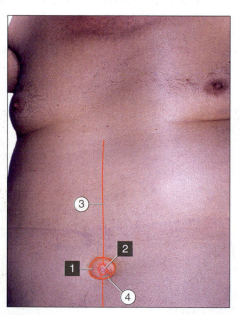

KEY
1 Extent of hernia sac
2 Paraumbilical defect
③ Linea alba
④ Umbilicus

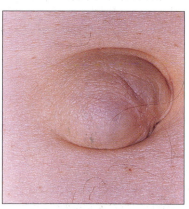

Fig. 7.6 Close up of paraumbilical hernia

Indirect and direct inguinal hernias

History

Patients often present with a groin lump that may be painless. Patients may also have a dragging sensation or tenderness in the inguinal area.

Ask about features that predispose to hernia formation:

- respiratory (chronic cough)
- gastrointestinal (constipation)
- genitourinary (prostatism)
- occupation (heavy lifting)
- previous surgery
- trauma
- collagen diseases.

Ask about features that will influence fitness for anaesthesia and surgery, and the approach used:

- cardiovascular disease
- respiratory conditions
- medications
- allergies
- past surgical history.

Examination of the groin for inguinal hernia

Exposure. Expose the abdomen, groin and external genitalia (Figs 7.7, 7.8, 7.9).

Positioning. Examine the patient while he is lying down with one pillow under the head, then when standing.

Inspection. Look for surgical scars, including laparoscopic scars. Ask the patient to cough and look for a visible cough impulse on each side. Remember the normal anatomy.

Palpation. Ask the patient if the hernia is tender.

Reduction. If the hernia does not reduce spontaneously on lying down, ask the patient if he can reduce the hernia. Gently use your fingers to help reduce the hernia.

Control points. It should be possible in most patients to differentiate between a direct (Fig. 7.8 **1b**) and an indirect **1a** inguinal hernia. With the hernia reduced, place two fingers firmly over the site of the deep inguinal ring (Fig 7.9 ⑦), ask the

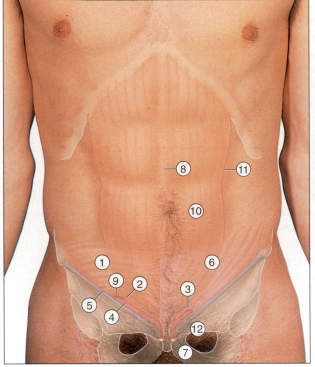

KEY
1. Internal oblique
2. Conjoint tendon
3. Superficial inguinal ring
4. Cremaster muscle
5. Inguinal ligament
6. Aponeurosis of external oblique
7. Spermatic cord
8. Linea alba
9. Deep inguinal ring
10. Rectus muscle
11. Rectus sheath
12. Pubic tubercle

Fig. 7.7 Normal anatomy of the lower abdominal wall

KEY
1a Indirect hernia sac
1b Direct hernia sac
2. Inferior epigastric artery
3. Femoral artery
4. Inguinal ligament
5. Spermatic cord
6. Testis
7. Pubic tubercle
8. Deep inguinal ring

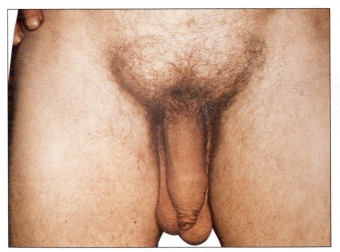

Fig. 7.8 Bilateral inguinal hernia

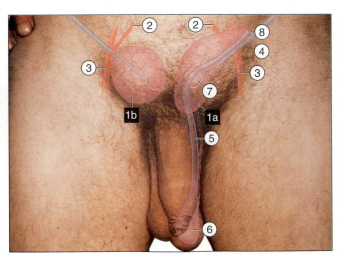

patient to cough; the fingers should prevent the hernia protruding along the inguinal canal if the hernia is an indirect hernia (Fig. 7.8 **1a** . If finger pressure over the deep inguinal ring fails to prevent the hernia protruding, reduce the hernia again, apply pressure over the position for a direct inguinal hernia **1b** and ask the patient to cough again. This should demonstrate control of a direct hernia.

Differentiating a hernia from a testicular swelling. An inguinal hernia protrudes from the deep inguinal ring (Fig. 7.10 ③) down the inguinal canal, passing medial to the pubic tubercle ⑦ (although a large hernia **1** may bulge over the tubercle hiding it, and down into the scrotum). To differentiate an inguinal hernia **1** from a testicular swelling or the testis ⑨ , feel above the lump ⑩ . If you can 'get above the lump' then it is related to the testis, its coverings or associated structures. If you cannot 'get above the lump', it is an inguinoscrotal (indirect) hernia **1** .

Percussion. Percussion is of limited value in the examination of a hernia. The note may be tympanic over a hernia containing bowel.

Auscultation. Auscultation may demonstrate bowel sounds.

Problems and pitfalls of examining the groin for hernias

- Scars hidden in skin creases or hair
- Obesity
- Previous surgery
- Other medical conditions (e.g. skin conditions).

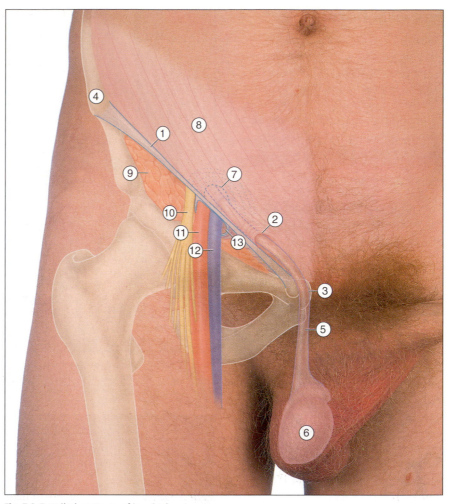

Fig. 7.9 Detailed anatomy of inguinal region

KEY
① Inguinal ligament
② Superficial inguinal ring
③ Pubic tubercle
④ Anterior superior iliac spine
⑤ Spermatic cord
⑥ Testis
⑦ Deep inguinal ring
⑧ Aponeurosis of external oblique
⑨ Iliopsoas muscle
⑩ Femoral nerve
⑪ Femoral artery
⑫ Femoral vein
⑬ Femoral canal

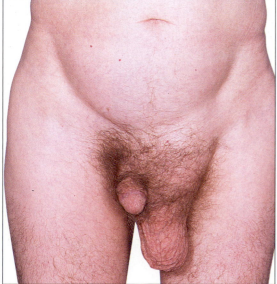

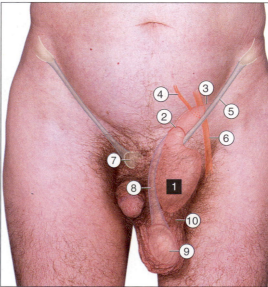

KEY
1 Indirect hernia
② External ring
③ Deep inguinal ring
④ Inferior epigastric artery
⑤ Inguinal ligament
⑥ Femoral artery
⑦ Pubic tubercle
⑧ Spermatic cord
⑨ Testis
⑩ Site to examine to distinguish indirect hernia from testicular swelling

Fig. 7.10 Inguinoscrotal hernia

Femoral hernias

History

Patients present with a lump that may be painless or tender. Most patients with a femoral hernia (Fig. 7.12) are elderly women.

In addition to general symptoms of hernia, ask about factors that pre-dispose to hernia formation:

- weight loss
- poor nutrition.

Ask about features that will influence fitness for anaesthesia and surgery, and the approach used.

Examination of the groin for femoral hernia

Exposure. Expose the abdomen, groin and external genitalia (Fig. 7.11). Examine patients while they are lying down with one pillow under the head, then when standing.

Inspection. Look for surgical scars including laparoscopic scars. Ask the patient to cough to elicit a cough impulse on each side (although a visible cough impulse is rarely seen in femoral hernia).

Palpation. Ask the patient if the hernia (Fig. 7.12 **1**) is tender.

Reduction. If the hernia does not reduce spontaneously on lying down, ask the patient if she can reduce the hernia. Gently use your fingers to help reduce the hernia. Larger hernias may not be reducible.

Control points. With the hernia reduced (if possible), place two fingers firmly over the femoral canal (Fig. 7.11 ④) lateral to the pubic tubercle ⑪ and medial to the femoral artery ② and the femoral vein ③. Ask the patient to cough; the fingers should prevent the hernia protruding.

Percussion. This is of limited value in the examination of a femoral hernia.

Auscultation may demonstrate bowel sounds, but is more useful if the patient has symptoms or signs of bowel obstruction when you examine the rest of the abdomen.

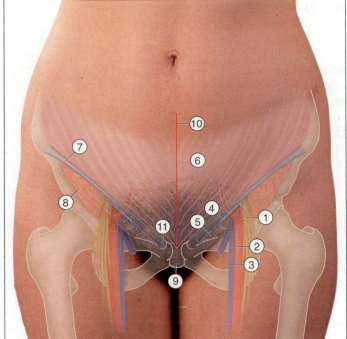

Fig. 7.11 Normal anatomy of femoral region

KEY
1. Femoral nerve
2. Femoral artery
3. Femoral vein
4. Femoral canal
5. Lacunar ligament
6. Aponeurosis of external oblique
7. Inguinal ligament
8. Iliopsoas muscle
9. Pubic symphysis
10. Midline
11. Pubic tubercle

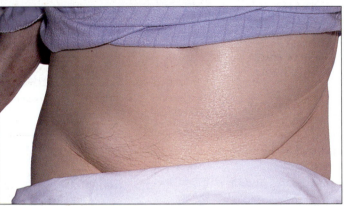

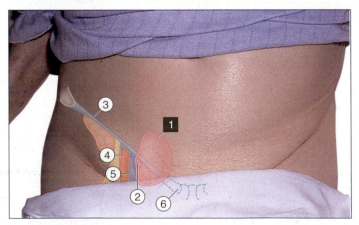

Fig. 7.12 Femoral hernia

KEY
1 Femoral hernia
2. Femoral canal
3. Inguinal ligament
4. Femoral artery
5. Femoral vein
6. Pubic tubercle

Unusual types of groin hernia

Pantaloon hernia

In addition to indirect inguinal hernia (Fig. 7.13 **2**), and direct inguinal hernia, a general weakness in the wall of the inguinal canal may result in in a pantaloon hernia **1** where there is herniation either side of the inferior epigastric artery ③ , said to look like pantaloon breeches.

KEY

1 Pantaloon hernia either side of inferior epigastric artery

2 Small indirect hernia

③ Inferior epigastric artery

④ Femoral artery

⑤ Inguinal ligament

⑥ Pubic tubercle

⑦ Anterior superior iliac spine

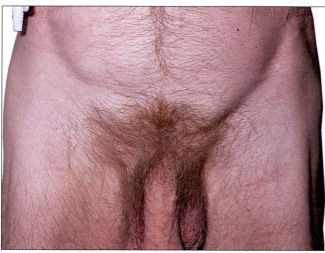
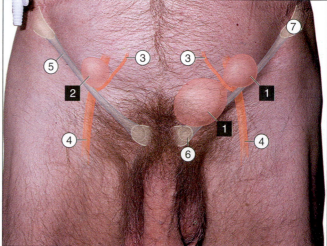

Fig. 7.13 Pantaloon hernia. Direct inguinal hernia plus indirect inguinal hernia in the same inguinal canal either side of the epigastric artery.

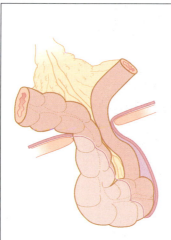
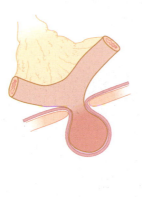
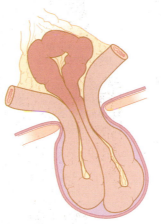
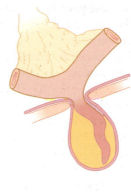

Fig. 7.14a Sliding hernia
When tissues that are normally extraperitoneal, such as the bladder or colon, form part of the wall of the hernial sac. It is thought that the extraperitoneal tissue slides down the canal pulling the peritoneum with it. The sac can contain other loops of bowel, and the portion of gut that forms the hernia wall can become strangled.

Fig. 7.14b Richter's hernia
Part of the bowel wall is caught in the hernia. If the sac is small, a small section of bowel wall can be caught and strangled without causing intestinal obstruction.

Fig. 7.14c Maydl's hernia
A rare variety of strangulation, when two loops of bowel are in the same sac. The intervening section of bowel in the abdomen is the first to suffer, and the strangulation is intra-abdominal.

Fig. 7.14d Littré's hernia
Strangulation of Meckel's diverticulum trapped in a hernial sac.

Other apects of hernias

Investigations for hernia

- Routine preoperative investigations:
  - full blood count
  - urea and electrolytes
  - ECG
  - chest radiograph (where appropriate)
- Herniography (Fig. 7.15) if the diagnosis is in doubt.

Differential diagnosis of groin hernias (Ch. 8)

- Lymph nodes
- Epididymal cyst
- Hydrocele
- Varicocele
- Testis swelling (tumours, ectopic)
- Lipoma
- Saphenovarix
- Skin lesions.

Surgery

The surgical treament of a hernia comprises inspecting then replacing the sac contents into the peritoneal cavity and repair of the hernial defect.

Complications of untreated hernia

- Pain
- Increasing size
- Ischaemia of contents
- Necrosis of contents
- Death.

Complications of hernia surgery

- Early:
  - urinary retention
  - spermatic cord/vascular damage
  - wound infection
  - chest infection
- Late:
  - hernia recurrence
  - testicular atrophy.

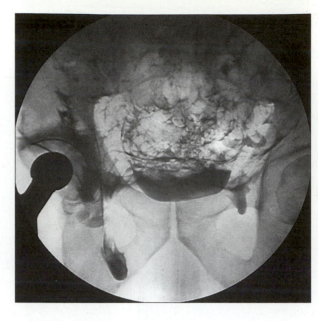

Fig. 7.15 Herniogram showing bilateral inguinal hernia (arrows)

Table 7.1 A summary of how to distinguish between inguinal and femoral hernia

	Indirect inguinal hernia	Direct inguinal hernia	Femoral hernia
Typical patient	Younger male	Older male	Old female
Proportion of groin hernias	60%	25%	15%
Anatomy	Commences at the deep ring, lateral to the inferior epigastric artery, and passes within the coverings of the spermatic cord	Bulges medial to the inferior epigastric artery	Emerges from the femoral canal
Relationship to the pubic tubercle	Starts lateral to and above the tubercle, but passes superomedial to the scrotum	Lies above the tubercle	Passes inferolateral to the tubercle
Descends into scrotum?	Yes	No	No
Obstructs or strangulates?	Yes	Rarely	Yes

8 Groin and scrotum

Lumps in the groin or scrotum can be divided into three categories: scrotal swellings, non-hernia groin lumps and hernias (Chapter 7). In addition, skin lesions (sebaceous cyst, squamous carcinoma of the penis) may occur in this region.

History

The age and sex of the patient are obviously crucial to the likely diagnosis. The history of the swelling – when it first appeared, whether it is tender, if it has changed in size, whether it can be moved, what structures it is attached to – is indicative of the likely diagnosis. Is there more than one lump? Are the lumps unilateral or bilateral?

Is there a history of trauma, recent exercise or previous surgery (especially hernia or scrotal surgery), or investigation such as femoral artery puncture (particularly for angiography)? Is there a history of sexually transmitted disease?

Past medical history, medications and systematic enquiry should also be documented.

Examination

Exposure. Full exposure of the groin area is necessary to ensure that the femoral triangles bounded by the inguinal ligament (Fig. 8.1 ④) adductor longus ⑧ and sartorius ⑨ are clearly visible and in the male that the external genitalia ⑤ ⑥ are visible. Particularly in males, hair or scrotal skin may obscure previous surgical scars and may make it difficult to see subtle changes in skin contour. Obese patients may hide abnormalities in the groin creases. Male patients should be asked to retract the foreskin (if present) to look for pathologies.

Inspection

Compare the right and left sides; look for swellings in the femoral triangles, scrotal swellings and any herniae. It is often easier to identify groin or scrotal swellings when the patient stands up;

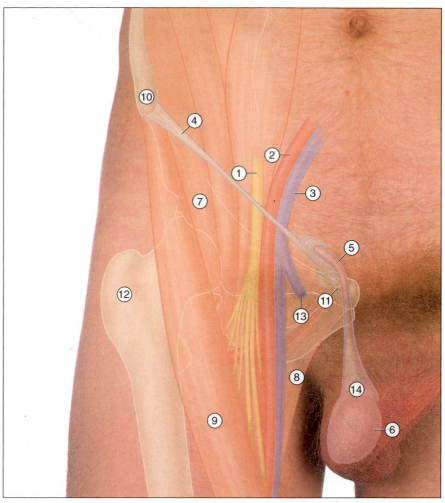

Fig. 8.1 Normal anatomy of the femoral triangle: vessels, nerves, testis and spermatic cord

KEY
① Femoral nerve
② Femoral artery
③ Femoral vein
④ Inguinal ligament
⑤ Spermatic cord
⑥ Testis
⑦ Iliacus muscle
⑧ Adductor longus muscle
⑨ Sartorius muscle
⑩ Anterior superior iliac spine
⑪ Pubic tubercle
⑫ Femur
⑬ Long saphenous vein
⑭ Epididymis

this is certainly the case for varicocele and herniae. Look for discoloration of the skin. Some groin swellings may be bilateral (e.g. lymph nodes, hernia).

Palpation

Ask the patient if there is any tenderness (tender areas should be palpated last if possible) and then gently palpate the groin, moving on to the scrotum. Again compare the left and right sides and confirm by palpation any abnormalities or differences visible on inspection.

On palpating the groin, identify whether the lump is single, multiple, unilateral or bilateral. Is the lump attached to the femoral artery ② or arising from a varicose long saphenous vein ⑬? What is the relationship of the lump or lumps to the femoral artery ② and inguinal ligament ④? Is the lump apparently fluctuant (suggesting a lipoma), expansile (suggesting a femoral artery aneurysm) or does it transmit a cough impulse (suggesting a saphenovarix)?

Palpation of the scrotum should compare sides, attempting to differentiate between the testis ⑥, epididymis ⑭ and cord ⑤ on each side. If a swelling is apparent, try to identify the structures to which it is attached (Fig. 8.2). Is the palpable lump truly scrotal – can one palpate above the lump and distinguish the palpable scrotal lump ⑥ ⑦ ⑧ ⑨ from an inguinoscrotal indirect inguinal hernia ①?

Transillumination of a fluid-filled scrotal swelling will identify whether it is a fluid collection and thus a hydrocele (Fig. 8.2 **6**), or solid **9** .

Auscultation

Auscultatation over a femoral artery ⑪ may reveal an arterial bruit, secondary to atherosclerotic arterial disease or an aneurysm **3** . Once again, compare the two sides. If a hernia is present **1** **2** , bowel sounds may be heard.

Investigation

Ultrasound is the key investigation to identify the precise anatomical position of the groin or scrotal lump relative to other structures, the contents of the lump, whether fluid (blood, hydrocele) or solid, the number of lesions and hence the probable diagnosis. Tumour markers (alpha fetoprotein (AFP) and human chorionic gonadotrophin (HCG)) are useful as disease markers for seminoma and teratoma of the testis.

Treatment

Treatment of groin swellings is either:
- expectant: leave alone; the problem is not causing distress, e.g. epididymal cyst, or will get better, e.g. lymphadenopathy secondary to viraemia
- surgical: biopsy, excise, repair or drain the abnormality.

Groin nodes

Groin nodes (Fig. 8.3) may be affected by primary or secondary conditions. The number, sites, duration and distribution of the nodes will suggest likely diagnoses.

Primary lymphadenopathy is caused by lymphoproliferative disorders. Secondary lymphadenopathy may result from:
- infection: bacterial, viral or other infective agent
- metastatic cancer from the lower limb, external genitalia (but not testes), anal region or a distant site.

History

A history suggestive of viral illness and multiple sites of lymphadenopathy may suggest the diagnosis. A careful history will elicit whether there is any primary lesion from which tumour may have metastasized and whether there are systemic symptoms such as sweating and fatigue.

Examination

On examination, the position and distribution, number, feel (firm, rubbery, shotty), size and tenderness of the nodes will be evident (Fig. 8.3 **1**). Any anatomical sites that the nodes may be draining should also be examined.

Investigation

A full blood count will identify any leucocytosis and if there is a lymphocytosis suggest a viral origin, which may be confirmed by performing viral titres. If malignancy is suspected, fine needle aspiration cytology of the node(s) can be performed to confirm the diagnosis. Excisional biopsy of one or more nodes may also be diagnostic.

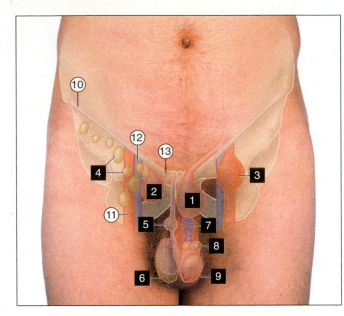

KEY
1 Indirect inguinal hernia
2 Femoral hernia
3 Femoral artery aneurysm
4 Lymph nodes
5 Cyst of cord
6 Hydrocele
7 Variocele
8 Epididymal cyst
9 Testicular cancer
⑩ Inguinal ligament
⑪ Femoral artery
⑫ Femoral vein
⑬ Pubic tubercule

Fig. 8.2 Groin and scrotal swellings

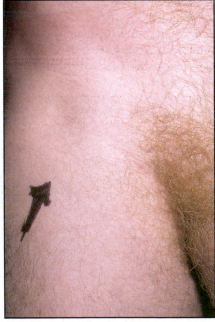

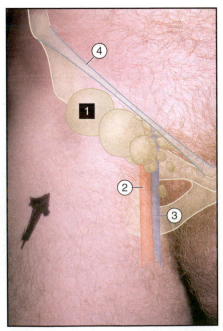

Fig. 8.3 Groin nodes

KEY
1 Lymph nodes
② Femoral artery
③ Femoral vein
④ Inguinal ligament

Testicular cancer

History

Testicular cancer is most common in the 20-to 40-year age group (teratoma peak age is 25, seminoma peak age is 35) as a progressive swelling (Fig. 8.4 **1**) which is usually painless and may be associated with a reactive hydrocele **2** .

Examination

On inspection, compare the left and right sides, looking for a difference in size (Fig. 8.4). Gently palpate the testes, normal side first. On the abnormal side, a palpable firm, symmetrically enlarged testis (or rarely an isolated nodule) may be evident **1** . However, a reactive hydrocele **2** around the testicular cancer may obscure the underlying testis. Clinical features which may be associated with a testicular tumour include gynaecomastia or an abdominal mass of retroperitoneal lymph nodes. The lymphatic drainage of the testes is to the para-aortic nodes due to the embryonic intra-abdominal origin of the testes, not to the groin, unlike other structures in the groin.

Investigation and treatment

On ultrasound scanning, the tumour **1** will be evident. An elevated AFP and/or HCG may support the diagnosis and can be useful to monitor disease burden. Following staging, which includes chest radiography and abdominal CT scanning to look for metastatic disease, surgical resection, radiotherapy and chemotherapy provide a high remission rate.

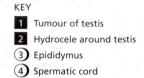

KEY
1 Tumour of testis
2 Hydrocele around testis
③ Epididymus
④ Spermatic cord

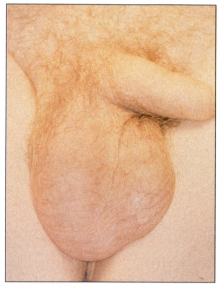

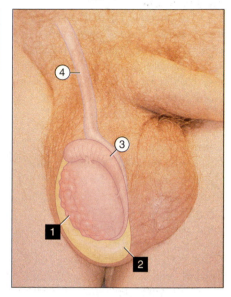

Fig. 8.4 Testicular cancer

Hydrocele

History

A hydrocele (Fig. 8.5 **1**) is sometimes secondary in response to trauma or an underlying abnormality of the testis (Fig. 8.4). Ask about recent trauma (most common in teenagers) or the development of a unilateral or bilateral swelling, often over several weeks.

Examination

Inspect the difference in size between the two sides, and palpate the hydrocele (Fig 8.5 **1**) to differentiate it from the cord ④ but note that the hydrocele may obscure the testis ② and epididymus ③ within. A hydrocele can be transilluminated by directing a torch light on to the skin overlying the hydrocele and looking for transilluminated light 'lighting up' the hydrocele.

Investigation and treatment

Ultrasound will demonstrate the hydrocele, testis and epididymus. Treatment, if required, is by drainage and then suturing the tunica to prevent reaccumulation of the fluid.

KEY
1 Hydrocele
② Testis
③ Epididymus
④ Spermatic cord

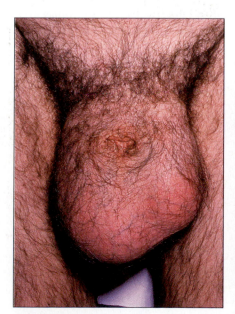

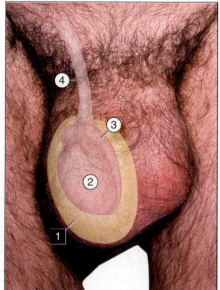

Fig. 8.5 Hydrocele

Torted testis

History

Testicular torsion (Fig. 8.6) usually occurs in pre-teenage boys and may occur following exercise. The testis **3** twists within the tunica vaginalis **2** because there is a free length of spermatic cord **1** within the tunica. Embryonic remnants such as a small cyst on the epididymus may twist and imitate testicular torsion. Clinically it may be impossible to distinguish between the two. There may have been a previous event of torsion causing extreme pain which resolved spontaneously. Abdominal pain may also be present owing to the embryological origin of the testes from within the abdomen.

Examination

The torted testis **3** lies higher and more horizontally in the scrotum and is often exquisitely tender, so examine the normal side first. As venous congestion of the torted testis worsens, the testis becomes more swollen and the skin overlying it may become reddened making it difficult to distinguish from epididymitis.

Investigations

Ultrasound may demonstrate the lack of blood flow to and from the testis and a reactive hydrocele.

Treatment

Surgery aims to untwist the torsion and then fix both testes with stitches so that they cannot tort once again. If the testis is black and necrotic at the time of surgery, orchidectomy is required on that side.

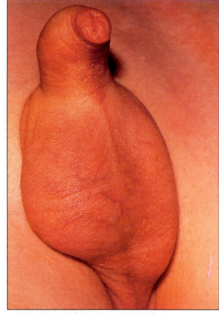

Fig. 8.6 Torted testis

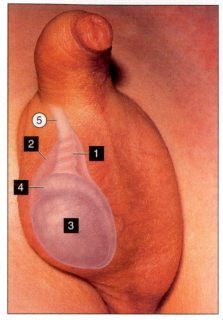

KEY

1 Torsion
2 High investment of tunica vaginalis
3 Ischaemic testis
4 Ischaemic epididymus
5 Spermatic cord

Varicocele

History

The patient may have noted some lumpiness or abnormal appearance of (or feel a heaviness in) the scrotum.

Examination

A varicocele (Fig. 8.7 **1**) is most obvious when the patient stands – the prominent veins, claimed to resemble a mass of worms, will be apparent. A varicocele is said to be more common on the left side, owing to the drainage of the left testicular vein into the left renal vein. Because of this venous drainage, a varicocele of recent onset may suggest a renal cancer.

Investigations and treatment

Investigation of the scrotum and the kidneys by ultrasound will demonstrate the multiple enlarged veins **1** travelling from the testis ② proximally around the spermatic cord. The veins can be ligated via an incision in the groin (or laparoscopically).

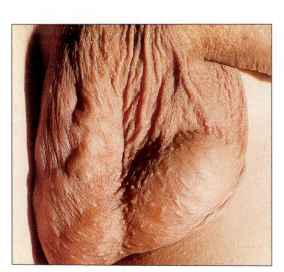

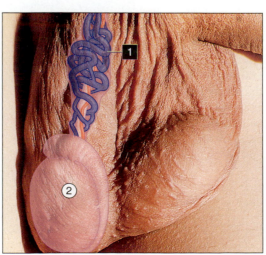

KEY

1 Varicocele
② Testis

Fig. 8.7 Varicocele

Groin infection

History
Cellulitis (Fig. 8.8 **2**), abscess or infected sebaceous cysts are comparatively common in the groin. The patient may be diabetic, have poor hygiene or inject drugs.

Examination
On inspection, look for the signs of acute inflammation **2** – redness, swelling (with associated tenderness and loss of function), a pointing abscess, any obvious breaches of the skin or lesions and any visible lymph nodes **1** . On gentle palpation, examine for lymph nodes, the extent of the tenderness and for crepitus due to gas-forming organisms. Mark the margin **2** of erythema (redness) with an indelible pen. This allows you to assess whether the cellulitis is spreading or regressing (responding to treatment).

Investigation and treatment
A raised white cell count may accompany systemic symptoms, and blood cultures may yield streptococci or staphylococci.

Treatment is by intravenous antibiotics with monitoring of the extent of the cellulitis **2** .

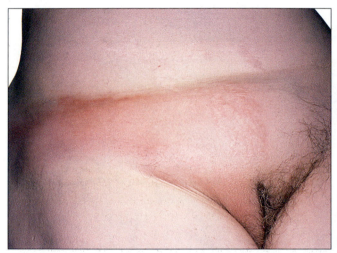

Fig. 8.8 Groin infection

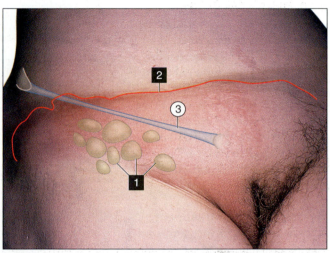

KEY
1 Lymph nodes
2 Cellulitis
③ Inguinal ligament

Femoral artery aneurysm

History

A femoral artery aneurysm (Fig. 8.9 **1**) usually follows arterial trauma (owing to arterial needle puncture) and more rarely atherosclerotic disease.

The patient may have had arterial puncture for angiography, so is likely to have a history of cardiovascular disease. The history should therefore include an assessment of cardiac and pulmonary systems, past medical history, and medications.

Examination

On inspection, the lump **1** lies below the mid-inguinal point (point midway between anterior superior iliac spine and symphysis pubis), where the external iliac becomes the femoral artery ②. The lump may show visible pulsation. On palpation, it is expansile; two fingers placed either side of the aneurysm are pushed away from each other by the expanding arterial wall. There may be a thrill due to blood flow and/or a bruit on auscultation.

Investigations and treatment

Investigation will include ultrasound scanning to delineate the extent of the aneurysm and treatment involves reconstruction of the abnormal segment of artery.

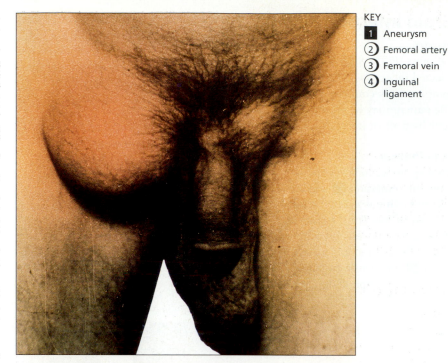

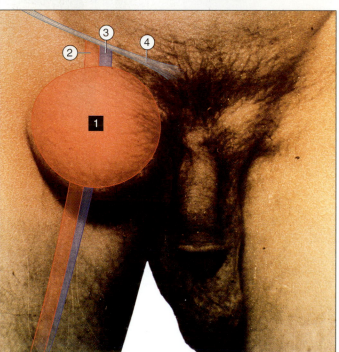

KEY

1 Aneurysm
② Femoral artery
③ Femoral vein
④ Inguinal ligament

Fig. 8.9 Femoral artery aneurysm

9 Lower limb

The arterial, venous, nervous and musculoskeletal systems of the lower limb are common sources of pathology. Arterial disease can be divided into occlusive, aneurysmal and fistula; venous disease into varicose veins and deep vein thrombosis.

Arterial disease

History

Age, smoking and diabetes are the three key predisposing factors to lower limb arterial disease.

A history of arterial insufficiency may include claudication, the onset of limb pain on exercise which is relieved by stopping. The claudication distance is the distance in yards or metres a person can walk before pain causes him or her to stop, and claudication distance may increase or decrease according to how severe the arterial insufficiency becomes.

Claudication occurs distal to the site of occlusive disease, so femoral ⑤ or popliteal ⑦ artery stenosis causes calf claudication, external iliac stenosis ② causes thigh/calf claudication and external ② plus internal ③ iliac insufficiency causes buttock, thigh and calf claudication. Bilateral lower limb claudication may be caused by aortic insufficiency. Rest pain signifies impending gangrene and commonly occurs when the patient is in bed at night, because of reduced perfusion pressure in the warm, horizontal lower limb; it can be relieved by lowering the limb over the side of the bed.

Acute arterial insufficiency results in pain, in a pallid, pulseless limb, and the limb is perishingly cold. With time, the limb becomes paraesthetic and powerless.

General medical history should include a history of smoking (current, previous, never, number of cigarettes) and diabetes, with a note of the type of diabetes and the degree of diabetic control. Ischaemic heart disease, cerebrovascular accidents, hyper-

tension, hypercholesterolaemia, rheumatic heart disease, family history of vascular disease or chronic obstructive pulmonary disease may be associated with lower limb arterial disease. The use of medication is important for control of cardiac disease, hypertension and diabetes.

Ask about the lifestyle effects of arterial disease including how it affects daily living and mobility.

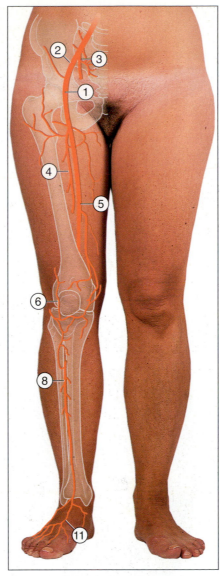

Fig. 9.1 Arteries of the lower limb

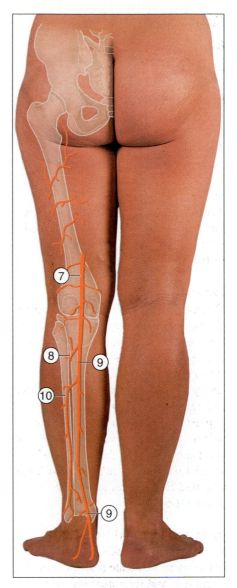

KEY
① Common femoral artery
② External iliac artery
③ Internal iliac artery
④ Deep femoral artery
⑤ Superficial femoral artery
⑥ Arterial network around knee
⑦ Popliteal artery
⑧ Anterior tibial artery
⑨ Posterior tibial artery
⑩ Peroneal artery
⑪ Dorsalis pedis artery

Examination

Patients should have both lower limbs exposed, wear brief underwear, and lie comfortably on a bed. Ensure that you can see both lower limbs and do not forget to expose and inspect pressure points such as the heel, lateral border of the foot, malleoli, first metatarsal head, between the toes and (when appropriate) underneath amputation stumps.

On **inspection**, look for chronic

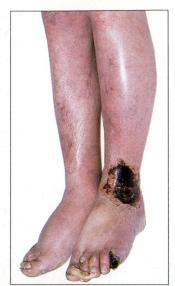
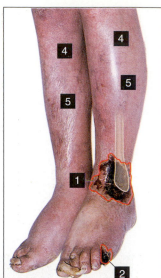
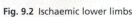

KEY

1. Arteriopathic ulcer
2. Gangrenous fifth toe
3. Demarcation of critrical ischaemia
4. Atrophic skin
5. Hair loss
6. Hyperaemia

Fig. 9.2 Ischaemic lower limbs

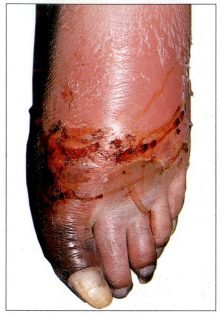
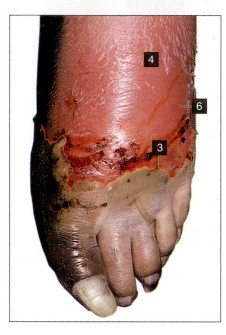

Fig. 9.3 Ischaemic foot

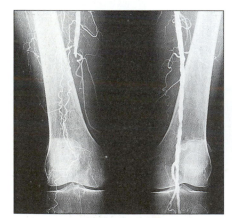

Fig. 9.4 Angiogram of lower limb arteries showing atherosclerotic disease

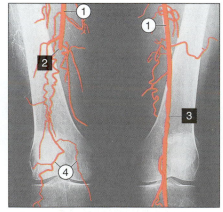

KEY

1. Femoral artery
2. Stenosis at hiatus in adductor magnus muscle
3. Atherosclerotic popliteal artery
4. Collateral vessels around knee

signs of ischaemia: shiny atrophic skin (Fig. 9.2 **4**), hair loss **5** , atrophic nails. Gangrene **2** , pallor of one limb or hyperaemic redness (Fig. 9.3 **6**), secondary to ischaemia, give an indication of the extent and severity of the ischaemia. Any amputation site and surgical scars should be examined and noted. Look for ulceration (Fig. 9.2 **1**), particularly over the pressure points and the lateral malleolus, gangrene **2** and any deformities or muscle wasting. Perform Buerger's test in which the lower limb is elevated, blanches and then becomes hyperaemic on resuming a dependent position.

Palpate the pulse for rate, rhythm and regularity and measure diastolic and systolic blood pressure on the upper limb. Using the dorsum of your fingers, compare the temperature to the two lower limbs; palpate for ankle oedema; test the nail bed for capillary refill time which should be no more than 2 seconds. Palpate the femoral pulses (Fig. 9.1 ①), in the groin at the midinguinal point, the popliteal arteries ⑦ (with the knee flexed to 90°), the posterior tibial artery ⑨ posterior to the medial malleolus and the dorsalis pedis pulses ⑪. The pulses should be recorded as 0 (absent), +/− (reduced), 1 (normal) or 2 (aneurysmal). Seek any evidence of radiofemoral delay secondary to co-arctation of the aorta.

Auscultation will demonstrate a bruit if there is abnormal flow but no bruit if there is no flow. Auscultation of the femoral arteries should be performed, comparing the two sides.

Investigation

Investigations include urine testing for glucose and protein (as a measure of diabetic control and renal disease), full blood count for anaemia, polycythemia, plasma viscosity/ESR (for arteritis), biochemistry for diabetic control, including haemoglobin A1, and renal function. An ECG and chest radiograph may demonstrate cardiac and respiratory disease. Pulse pressures using Doppler scanning document the extent of lower limb disease (ankle: brachial pressure index) and angiography (Fig. 9.4) and angioscopy provide a roadmap of the sites of atherosclerotic arterial disease. In the lower limb, the hiatus in adductor magnus where the femoral artery becomes the popliteal artery is a common site of stenosis (Fig. 9.4 **2**).

Management

The management of lower limb ischaemia usually occurs over several years.

Conservative measures. Control of diabetes mellitus, encouraging exercise, foot and skin care and stopping smoking all reduce progress of atherosclerotic disease.

Medical. Optimize medical therapy for diabetes and cardiopulmonary disease to maximize tissue delivery of oxygen.

Surgical. For acute ischaemia, treat with streptokinase or use a Fogarty balloon to retrieve thrombus. For chronic ischaemia, treat by angioplasty with balloon dilation or stent. Reconstructive surgery to restore flow beyond stenotic segments, sympathectomy for symptom relief or amputation of severely ischaemic tissue may be required. Digital amputation (Fig. 9.5), below knee (BK) amputation (Fig. 9.6) and above knee (AK) amputation (Fig. 9.7) are most commonly performed.

Rehabilitation

Following angioplasty, reconstructive surgery and particularly amputation, restoring mobility (including the use of sticks, prosthesis or wheelchair) and everyday functional living are high priorities.

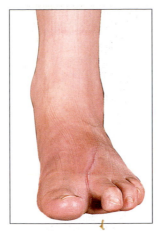
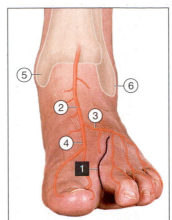

KEY
1 Scar from second digit amputation
2 Dorsalis pedis artery
3 Arcuate artery
4 Communication with deep plantar artery
5 Medial malleolus
6 Lateral malleolus

Fig. 9.5 Digital amputation

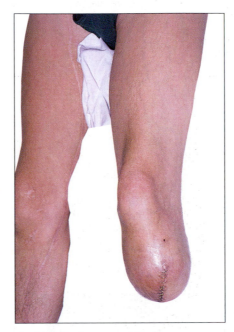

Fig. 9.6 Below knee amputation

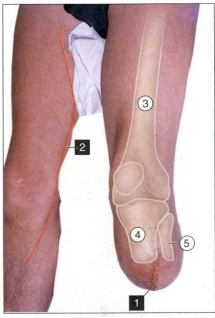

KEY
1 Amputation scar
2 Scars from contralateral arterial reconstruction
3 Femur
4 Tibia
5 Fibula

KEY
1 Amputation scar
2 Femur
3 Superficial femoral artery
4 Deep femoral artery

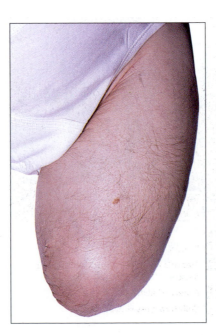

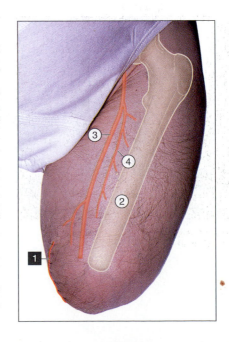

Fig. 9.7 Above knee amputation

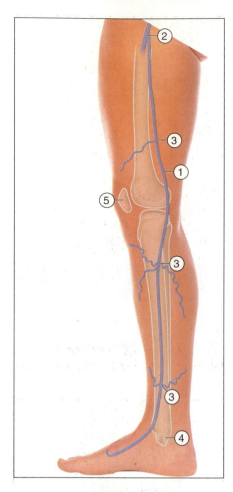

KEY
1. Great saphenous vein
2. Saphenofemoral junction
3. Common sites of incompetent perforating veins
4. Medial malleolus
5. Patella

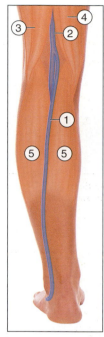

KEY
1. Short saphenous vein
2. Popliteal vein
3. Biceps femoris muscle
4. Semitendinosus muscle
5. Gastrocnemius muscle

Fig. 9.9 Normal anatomy of the short saphenous vein

Fig. 9.8 Normal anatomy of the great saphenous vein

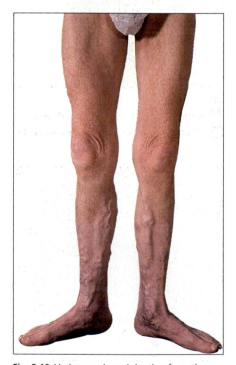

Fig. 9.10 Varicose veins originating from the great saphenous system

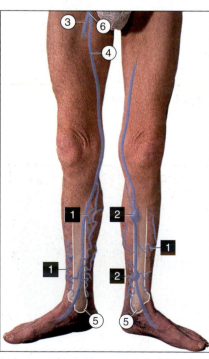

KEY
1. Varicose veins
2. Incompetent perforators
3. Femoral vein
4. Great saphenous vein
5. Medial malleolus
6. Saphenofemoral junction

Venous disease of the lower limb

History

The history should include the age and sex of the patient, the symptoms, their duration, and the distribution of the varicose veins. The onset may be following a deep venous thrombosis or trauma to the lower limb or be exacerbated by pregnancy; more commonly, varicose veins arise from congenital valve defects at the sapheno-femoral junction (Fig. 9.8 ②), of the short saphenous system (Fig. 9.9) or of perforating veins (Fig. 9.8 ③). Ask if varicose veins affect one or both lower limbs and which parts of the limbs are involved. Symptoms include unsightly distended veins (Fig. 9.10 **1**), skin itch, skin discoloration (Fig. 9.11 **3**), lipodermosclerosis and ulceration (Fig. 9.12 **2** **1**). A vague ache sometimes attributed to varicose veins may not be improved by surgery. A history of previous treatments for the varicose veins, including conservative measures and surgery, should be elicited.

Examination

Both lower limbs should be exposed up to the groin and the patient examined standing (Fig. 9.10).

On **inspection**, compare right and left sides. Note the anatomical course of the great saphenous (Figs 9.8 ①, 9.10 ④) and the short saphenous (Fig. 9.9 ①) veins. Inspect for surgical scars, which in the groin may be quite difficult to see but should be related to the distribution of the superficial veins of the lower limbs. Look for varicosities, particularly at the sites of perforators (Fig. 9.10 **2**), skin discoloration, lipodermosclerosis and even ulceration around the ankle.

On **palpation**, feel the soft bluish reducible swelling of the veins (Fig. 9.10 **1** **2**), particularly at the sapheno-femoral junction ⑥ and along the course of the great saphenous vein ④. On asking the patient to cough, a fluid thrill may be evident at the incompetent saphenofemoral junction. The varicosities will empty on direct pressure. Defects in the fascia at perforation sites **2** may also be palpable.

It is important to check the arterial pulses of the lower limb for coexisting arterial disease and to be aware that there are other causes of leg ulcers – arteriopathy, neuropathy, diabetic, vasculitic (rheumatoid arthritis), infective and malignancy.

On **percussion** over the great saphenous vein below the knee, the transmitted pressure wave should be detected all the way up the column of blood in the varicose vein to the saphenofemoral junction proximally.

The Trendelenburg test is designed to identify the level of incompetent perforators (Figs 9.8 ③, 9.10 ②) – ask the patient to lie flat, then elevate one lower limb and empty the veins manually. Place a tourniquet around the upper thigh, distal to the sapheno-femoral junction (Figs 9.8 ②, 9.10 ⑥), and with the tourniquet pressure applied ask the patient to stand. If there is saphenofemoral incompetence alone, the varicose veins do not refill until you release the tourniquet. If there are incompetent perforators distally (Fig. 9.10 ②) the varicose veins will fill through the perforators. The Trendelenburg test may be repeated more distally to identify the perforators on both the lower limbs.

Investigations

Investigations include a full blood count, urea and electrolytes, ECG and chest X-ray to determine fitness for anaesthesia. Doppler scanning (Fig. 9.13) can be used to identify perfor-ators with a blood flow from the high-pressure deep system to the low-pressure superficial varicose system via incompetent valves. Ascending phlebography is useful, particularly if there is a history of deep venous thrombosis.

Management

Graduated compression stockings, injections with sclerosant (below the knee), laser therapy or local ligation for minor varicose veins; sapheno-femoral (high) ligation, stripping out the great saphenous vein from the groin to just below the knee and multiple ligations or avulsions of other varicosities constitute the surgical treatment options. Skin grafts may be required for varicose ulceration.

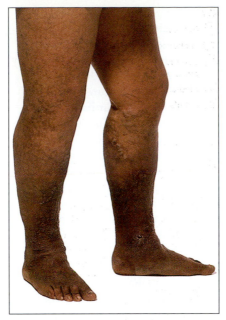

Fig. 9.11 Varicose veins from the great saphenous vein (advanced disease) with bilateral skin changes

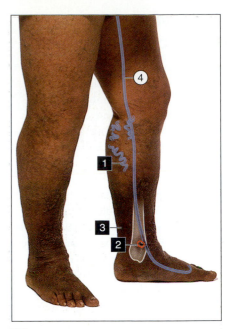

KEY

1 Varicosities	3 Skin discoloration
2 Varicose ulcer	④ Great saphenous vein

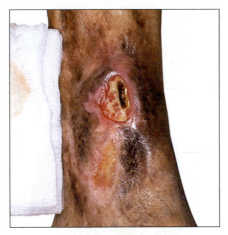

Fig. 9.12 Varicose ulcer

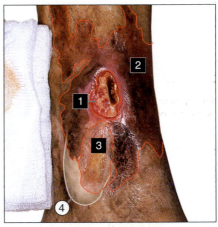

KEY

1 Ulcer	3 Healed ulcer
2 Lipodermosclerosis	④ Medial malleolus

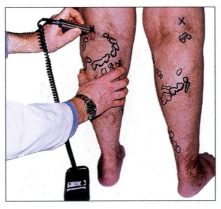

Fig. 9.13 Varicose veins from short saphenous system. Doppler probe and calf compression in use to show site of deep to superficial incompetence (marked X)

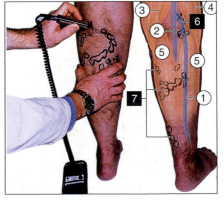

KEY

① Short saphenous vein	⑤ Gastrocnemius muscle
② Popliteal vein	6 Incompetent popliteal/short saphenous communicating
③ Semitendinosus muscle	
④ Biceps muscle	7 Varicosities

Deep venous thrombosis

Deep venous thrombosis (DVT) should be distinguished from other causes of a swollen limb, including cardiovascular (chronic cardiac failure), renal (nephrotic syndrome) and low protein (hypoalbuminaemia).

History

Ask about predisposing factors, which include immobility, old age, pelvic, abdominal or lower limb (particularly hip) surgery or trauma, or malignancy. Ask about the lower limb swelling, whether its onset has been sudden or gradual and whether it is increasing. Is the limb tender (as it often is) and reducing mobility (Fig. 9.15)? Ask about respiratory symptoms (which may reflect pulmonary embolic disease): sharp pleuritic chest pain, particularly on inspiration, and more rarely shortness of breath or haemoptysis. A past medical history should include previous venous thromboses, pulmonary embolism or lower limb or pelvic trauma, smoking and medications (such as tamoxifen) which may be associated with increased risk of DVT.

Examination

The lower limbs should be exposed to the groin and the patient asked if the limbs are tender.

On **inspection**, compare the right with the left side and the distribution of the swelling. Does it affect the foot and calf (Fig. 9.14), the thigh as well, or the whole lower limb (Fig. 9.15)? Is it unilateral or bilateral? Look at the colour of the limb (Fig. 9.15 **2** **3**), and whether the skin looks swollen **1** and shiny **4** .

The post-thrombotic limb may show chronic lower limb swelling, dilated or varicose veins, varicose eczema and even ulceration.

On gentle **palpation**, look for pitting oedema and measure the size of the calf and thigh 10 cm below the tibial tuberosity and 10 cm above the

top of the patella, comparing the left side with the right side. The side with a thrombosis should be enlarged but such measurements may not show any difference and are not diagnostic. Check for a temperature difference using the back of your hand, comparing the right and left sides (the thrombosed side should be warmer).

Examine the respiratory system, seeking evidence of embolism with secondary infarction of pulmonary segments, for which the signs including a pleural rub may be evident.

Investigations

Doppler scanning for deep venous thrombosis is a non-invasive but less specific method than ascending venography (Fig. 9.16) to define the extent of the venous thrombosis, i.e. whether it affects the calf, thigh and/or pelvic veins **1** . Other investigations include chest X-ray, which may be abnormal if a pulmonary embolism has occurred and an ECG may show signs of right heart strain.

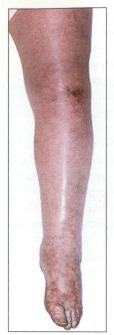 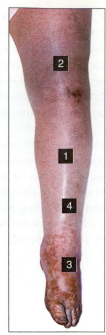

Fig. 9.15 Deep venous thrombosis – advanced disease

KEY

1 Swollen
2 Bluish
3 Mottled
4 Shiny skin

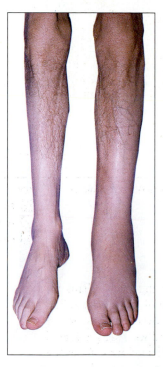

Fig. 9.14 Unilateral deep venous thrombosis

A perfusion scan may show segmental defects and, particularly if matched with a ventilation scan, can provide low, medium or high suspicion of venous pulmonary embolism. The definitive investigation, although rarely performed, is pulmonary angiography.

Management includes the use of graduated compression stockings and heparin (with subsequent conversion to warfarin); extensive or recurrent thromboses may be treated by a venacaval filter to prevent fatal pulmonary embolism.

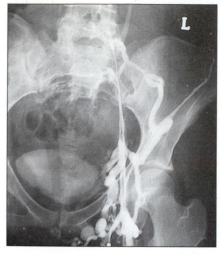

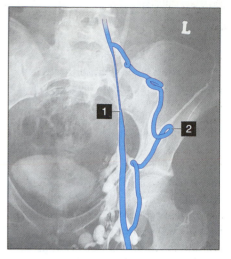

Fig. 9.16 Venogram of deep ileofemoral venous thrombosis

KEY

| 1 | Thrombus occluding external iliac vein |
| 2 | Collateral venous circulation |

Lymphoedema

Lower limb lymphoedema may be primary, owing to failure of lymphatic channel development, or secondary to lymphatic obstruction, usually in the groin or pelvis, commonly by tumour or infectious organisms.

History

Ask about the onset, severity and progression of the swelling, a past history of malignant disease or travel to tropical climates.

Examination

On **inspection**, assess the side(s) involved (Fig. 9.17) and the extent and severity of the lymphoedema (to knee, thigh or buttock). Look for ulceration, skin thickening or infection of the lymphoedematous limb.

Investigation

This aims to differentiate lymphoedema from deep venous thrombosis and identify the cause. Lymphangiography and CT scan of the pelvis (for secondary lymphoedema) should define the extent of the underlying problem and may identify the precipitating cause.

Management

Similar principles of management are used for lower limb lymphoedema as

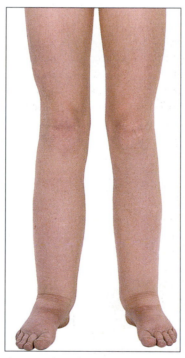

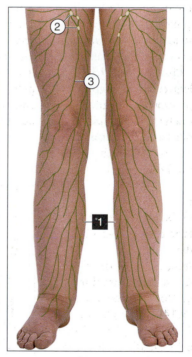

Fig. 9.17 Bilateral lymphoedema of lower limbs

KEY

1	Bilateral lymophoedema
2	Lymph nodes
3	Lymph vessels

for upper limb lymphoedema (see page 32, Fig. 4.17). The condition may be inproved by massage, limb elevation and wearing graduated compression stockings. As in the upper limb, skin care is important because poor lymphatic drainage can make infections (streptococcal and staphylococcal) difficult to treat.

Dropped foot

A dropped foot (Fig. 9.18: inability to dorsiflex the ankle) is secondary to peroneal nerve damage, either where the common peroneal nerve passes round the neck of the fibula (owing to trauma or pressure during surgery under anaesthesia) or from ischaemic necrosis as part of compartment syndrome.

History

Ask when the dropped foot was noted in relation to lower limb ischaemia, surgery or trauma. Has the dropped foot recovered at all?

Examination

On **inspection**, look for the classic position of the affected limb **2** and signs of the cause more proximally. The patient will be unable to flex the ankle and there may be associated altered sensation over the dorsum of the first interdigital space (Fig. 9.19 ③). If asked to walk, the high-stepping gait and downward slap of the affected limb are classic. A splint may be useful while any nerve regeneration occurs.

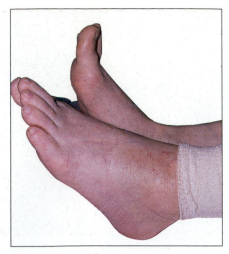
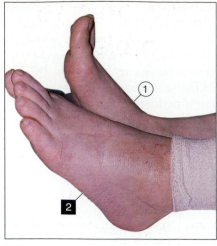

Fig. 9.18 Dropped foot

KEY
① Dorsiflexion of normal foot and great toe
2 Unable to dorsiflex foot or great toe

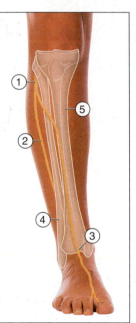

KEY
① Common peroneal nerve next to neck of fibula
② Deep peroneal nerve (motor)
③ Superficial peroneal nerve (sensory)
④ Fibula
⑤ Tibia

Fig. 9.19 Course of common, deep and superficial nerves

10 Skin and nails

History

The features of a lump wherever it lies in the body include:
- the duration of the lump
- whether the lump is tender
- any change in size, shape or colour
- any other lesions
- any associated features (pain, discharge)
- any predisposing events (e.g. insect bites).

Examination

On **inspection**, look for:
- the number (single/multiple)
- position
- size (in cm)
- shape
- colour
- outline of the margin
- contour of the surface
- any punctum.

After checking that it is not too painful, **palpate** the lesion.
- Is it hard or soft?
- Is it fluctuant? – use two fingers positioned on either side of the lump to detect fluctuance and a third to press on the lump.
- What is the relationship to the overlying skin – is the skin immobile over the lump (sebaceous cyst, Fig. 10.1) or can the skin be moved over the lump (lipoma, Fig. 10.2)?

Examine the regional lymph nodes.

Based on these features (Table 10.1), it should be possible to decide whether a lump is likely to be a sebaceous cyst, lipoma or lymph node (see Chapters 2 and 8).

Treatment

The lesion may be excised if troublesome, or left alone.

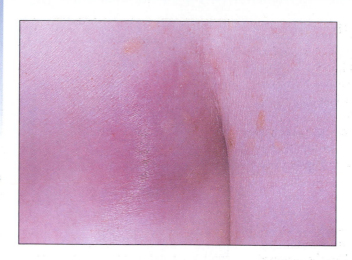

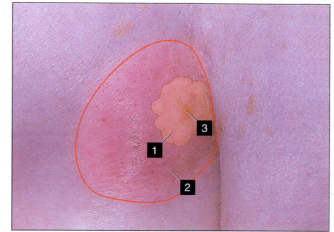

KEY

1	Sebaceous cyst
2	Erythema
3	Punctum

Fig. 10.1 Sebaceous cyst

Sebaceous cyst

There has usually been a long-standing scalp, neck, groin or axillary lump (Fig. 10.1 **1**) of about 1 cm which can fluctuate in size and may discharge cheesy material intermittently or become infected with erythema **2** and tenderness of the surrounding skin.

The punctum **3**, if visible, is a telltale sign; however, it may not be obvious. A sebaceous cyst **1** lies anatomically within the skin so the skin cannot be moved over the lump, in contrast to a lipoma. A sebaceous cyst may be excised if symptomatic or infected.

Table 10.1 Features of common lumps		
	Sebaceous cyst	**Lipoma**
Size	5 mm–2 cm	1–10 cm +
Shape	Spherical	Disc
Colour	May be red	Normal skin
Consistency	Soft or hard	Soft/fluctuant
Position	Scalp/axilla/neck	Trunk/limbs
Fixation	To skin	? To muscle
Associated features	Punctum Cheesy exudate	

Lipoma

A lipoma (Fig. 10.2) may be solitary or there may be multiple lipomata on the trunk or limbs.

On examination, note the features of the lump; a lipoma lies in the subcutaneous tissues and thus the skin can be moved over it (and it lacks a punctum). In addition, a lipoma may appear to be fluctuant, since fat is semiliquid at body temperature.

A lipoma ranges in size from 1 to 10 cm or more and may pass between muscle fascia planes so appearing attached to the underlying muscle. Rarely, lipomata are tender and even less commonly may be confused with a liposarcoma which is usually larger and fixed to the surrounding tissues.

The lipoma may be excised if symptomatic.

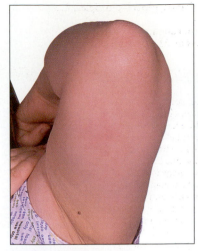
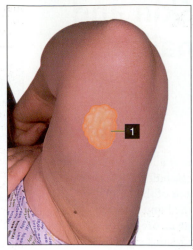

Fig. 10.2 Lipoma

KEY

1 Lipoma

Toenails

Ingrowing toenail (IGTN)

Usually the big toe (sometimes both) of a young adult male is affected, with the edges of the nail biting into the adjacent pulp tissue (Fig. 10.3 1) causing pain, inflammation 2 and sometimes superimposed infection 2 . On inspection, the ingrowing nail will be apparent 1 , together with signs of inflammation 2 (red, swollen, painful to touch) or infection (the addition of pus exuding from the nail).

Treatment may be by trimming the nail perpendicular to the direction of growth (incorrect trimming 3 may result in an IGTN). Excision of a wedge of the lateral edge of the nail or excision of the whole nail bed following avulsion of the nail are other surgical options.

Onychogryphosis (Fig. 10.4)

This is usually found in the elderly and is an overgrowth of the great toe (or other) nail(s) which comes to resemble a horn.

Treatment is by trimming the nail or avulsion.

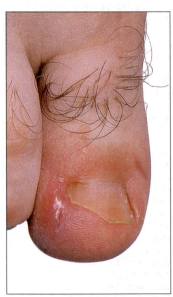
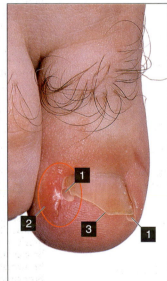

KEY

1 Ingrowing nail
2 Inflamed skin
3 Incorrectly trimmed nail

Fig. 10.3 Ingrowing toenail

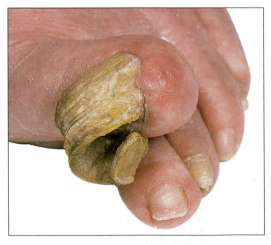

Fig. 10.4 Onychogryphosis

Index